Adult and Pediatric Spinal Deformities - Recent Advances and Evolution of Technologies

Edited by Mick Perez-Cruet and Lee-Onn Chieng

Published in London, United Kingdom

Adult and Pediatric Spinal Deformities - Recent Advances and Evolution of Technologies
http://dx.doi.org/10.5772/intechopen.111257
Edited by Mick Perez-Cruet and Lee-Onn Chieng

Contributors
Alexander V. Gubin, Alexey A. Kalashnikov, Alysha Jamison, Andrew Clarke, Dmitry Y. Zinenko, Evgenia M. Berdichevskaya, Hossein Nematian, Ilkhom E. Khujanazarov, Justin Scheer, Kathryn Park, Lee-Onn Chieng, Lee A. Tan, Mick Perez-Cruet, Mohammad Hossein Nabian, Olga M. Sergeenko, Pablo Pazmiño, Rouzbeh Motiei-Langroudi, Saeed Abdollahifard, Saeed Reza Mehrpour, Samer G. Zammar, Sergey O. Ryabykh, Shaker Barker, Timur A. Dzhumatov, Uduak-Obong I. Ekanem, Vladimir S. Klimov, Wei Tan, Weiye Zhang, Young Lee, Zahra Vahdati

First published in London, United Kingdom, 2024 by IntechOpen
IntechOpen is the global imprint of INTECHOPEN LIMITED, registered in England and Wales, registration number: 11086078, 167-169 Great Portland Street, London, W1W 5PF, United Kingdom

British Library Cataloguing-in-Publication Data
A catalogue record for this book is available from the British Library

Additional hard and PDF copies can be obtained from orders@intechopen.com

Adult and Pediatric Spinal Deformities - Recent Advances and Evolution of Technologies
Edited by Mick Perez-Cruet and Lee-Onn Chieng
p. cm.
Print ISBN 978-0-85466-353-8
Online ISBN 978-0-85466-352-1
eBook (PDF) ISBN 978-0-85466-354-5

For EU product safety concerns:
IN TECH d.o.o., Prolaz Marije Krucifikse Kozulić 3, 51000 Rijeka, Croatia,
info@intechopen.com or visit our website at intechopen.com.

Meet the editors

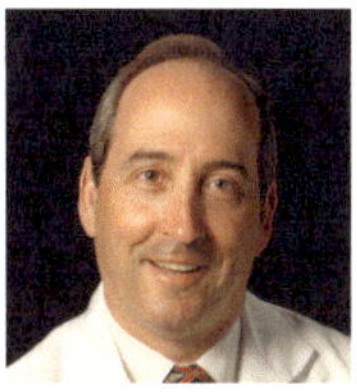

Dr. Mick Perez-Cruet is an internationally recognized pioneer in the treatment of spinal disorders using minimally invasive surgical techniques. His experience spans more than 30 years. He is vice chairman and professor in the Department of Neurosurgery, Oakland University William Beaumont School of Medicine, Michigan, USA. He is one of the core faculty for the ACGME Neurosurgery Residency Program at the same university and director of the Minimally Invasive Spine Fellowship Program. He is the Beaumont Neurosurgeon Champion for the Michigan Spine Surgery Improvement Collaborative (MSSIC), which is the largest comprehensive spine surgery outcome registry in the country. He is the founder and president of his practice Michigan Minimally Invasive Neurosurgical Institute, Michigan, USA. He dedicates much of his time to teaching neurosurgeons, fellows, residents, and medical students. He has served as the Michigan delegate to the Council of State Neurosurgical Societies (CSNS) for more than 20 years, was president of the Michigan Association of Neurological Surgeons (MANS), and holds several administrative positions within Corewell Health, East. Additionally, he is the president and founder of the Minimally Invasive Neurosurgical Society (MINS), a nationally recognized organization that promotes improved patient outcomes through surgeon teaching, cadaveric labs, and research to promote minimally invasive spine and cranial procedures.

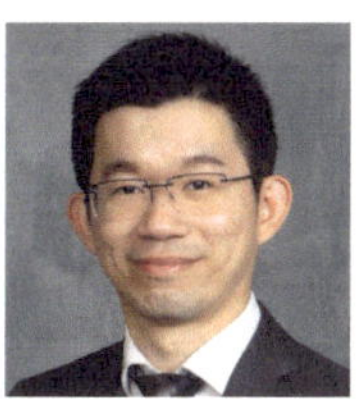

Dr. Lee-Onn Chieng is a neurosurgeon at Beaumont Health, Royal Oak, Michigan, USA. He received his MD from the University of Miami Miller School of Medicine, Florida, USA. In 2018 and 2020, Dr. Chieng received the Charles Kuntz Scholar Award (Top 20 Spine Abstract) from the American Association of Neurological Surgeons/Congress of Neurological Surgeons (AANS/CNS) Joint Spine Section on Disorder of the Spine and Peripheral Nerves. He also won the 2017 Stewart Dunsker Award from the AANS. He is interested in advancing the treatment of pediatric and adult spinal deformities.

Contents

Preface

In an era where patients seek not only efficacy but also enhanced recovery and minimal disruption to their lives, minimally invasive techniques emerge as a beacon of hope. Through meticulous planning, advanced imaging, and innovative instrumentation, these approaches offer the promise of smaller incisions, reduced tissue trauma, and accelerated recovery.

This book serves as a comprehensive guide, offering a deep dive into the multiple aspects of spinal deformities. From the fundamental principles to cutting-edge surgical techniques, readers will find a wealth of information to enhance their understanding and clinical practice.

As editors, it is our privilege to present this comprehensive guide, offering a panoramic view of traditional and minimally invasive strategies for spinal deformity correction. From the foundational principles to the intricacies of surgical techniques, each chapter serves as a roadmap for navigating the complexities of spinal deformity management with finesse and precision.

We extend our deepest gratitude to the contributors whose dedication and expertise have made this book possible. It is our hope that this compilation of chapters will serve as an invaluable resource for surgeons, residents, and allied healthcare professionals, empowering them to embrace the future of spinal deformity care with confidence and proficiency.

Lee-Onn Chieng and Mick Perez-Cruet
Department of Neurosurgery,
Corewell Health Beaumont University Hospital,
USA

Chapter 1

Treating Lumbar Scoliosis with Single-Level Minimally Invasive Transforaminal Lumbar Interbody Fusion

Mick Perez-Cruet and Lee-Onn Chieng

Abstract

Substantial evidence exists supporting lumbar fusion procedures in cases of spondylolysis, spondylolisthesis, and other cases of sagittal deformity. However, coronal deformity can also be a cause of low back and leg pain. One hundred seven patients underwent minimally invasive transforaminal lumbar interbody fusion (MITLIF). All patients had preoperative and postoperative radiographs exhibiting a clear coronal deformity that correlated with their symptomatology. Dynamic radiographs were analyzed using a three-point angle measurement tool through the EasyViz viewer program. Pre-op and post-op Cobb angles (CA) were recorded along with Health-related Quality of Life (HRQL) measures, Visual Analog Scale, Oswestry Disability Index, and SF-36. The average CA decreased from 9.47 pre-op to 7.54 post-op ($p < 0.05$). CA ranged from 0.7 to 43.2% pre-op, and 0.7 to 34.1% post-op. There was a statistically significant ($p < 0.05$) correlation between CA improvement and HRQL measure improvement. There has not been an appropriate level of focus on coronal deformity, its relationship to HRQL measures, and long-term prognosis. In our study, CA was reduced by 21% on average with just a single-level fusion, supporting the consideration of a focused single-level fusion versus a large multilevel fusion in cases of coronal deformity, especially in elderly patients.

Keywords: pain, spine and spinal disease, scoliosis, minimally invasive, surgery

1. Introduction

Spinal deformity is defined by malalignment in curvature of one or more levels of the vertebral column. Spinal deformities involve the combination of sagittal, coronal, and axial planes [1]. Major developments in spinal deformity correction techniques did not occur until 1940–1970 when poliomyelitis was an epidemic causing patients to suffer from excruciating pain due to abnormal spine curvature and associated cardiopulmonary compromise, ultimately leading to an untimely death [2].

 IntechOpen

The Harrington procedure was a novel technique at the time and involved placement of hooks on the bony architecture of posterior elements that were attached to stainless steel rods, this technique launched the idea of utilizing internal stabilization to correct spinal deformity, which prior to that time relied mainly on casting and external stabilization techniques [3]. The advent of polyaxial head pedicle screws advanced techniques for scoliotic spinal deformity treatment by allowing the placement of rods even when the pedicles are misaligned and utilization of these screws alone or in combination with proximal hook instrumentation was revealed to yield a significant improvement in primary and secondary curve correction in idiopathic thoracic scoliosis [4, 5]. Adult spinal deformity (ASD) most often occurs because of wear- and tear-associated degeneration that accumulates over time, which is why it is so prevalent in the elderly population. Studies have documented the importance of sagittal deformity correction and significant improvement in health-related quality of life (HRQOL) measures [6, 7]. Sagittal imbalance can lead to progressive deformity, strain on paraspinal musculature, ligamentous and joint hypertrophy, spinal stenosis, spondylolisthesis, and even problems with social interactions due to the inability of horizontal gaze maintenance [8, 9]. These resultant conditions often have a disastrous impact on the patient's ability to ambulate and carry out activities of daily living (ADL). Scoliosis, which is typically defined by an abnormality of spinal curvature in the coronal plane, commonly occurs due to aging-related collapse of intervertebral disks and vertebral body compression fractures that result in exaggeration or deficiency of normal curvatures of the spine [10]. Unfortunately, an insufficient amount of data is available regarding the outcomes of coronal deformity correction with minimally invasive spinal procedures. Therefore, we undertook the challenge to provide long-term data on radiographic and clinical outcomes of corrective surgery performed on individuals suffering from coronal deformity-associated pathology.

2. Materials and methods

The study was designed to follow a consecutive series of patients over an extended period to examine radiographic and clinical measures of surgical success. Three hundred fifty patients who underwent minimally invasive transforaminal lumbar interbody fusion (MI-TLIF) were followed for seven consecutive years. All of the procedural outcomes and test results analyzed were previously collected as part of the course of routine treatment, no additional interventions were required, and data analysis did not involve use of subject identifiers, thereby waiving the need for informed consent. The data was pared down to 107 patients who had preoperative and postoperative radiographs that exhibited a clear coronal deformity that correlated with the patient's symptomatology. A detailed description of our MI-TLIF approach can be found in our previous investigation entitled "Complication management with minimally invasive spine procedures" [11]. Dynamic radiographs were analyzed using a three-point angle measurement tool through the EasyViz viewer program. Cobb angles were recorded preoperatively and postoperatively along with a validated full set of Health-related Quality of Life (HRQOL) measures, such as Short Form-36 (SF-36), as well as the Visual Analog Scale (VAS) and Oswestry Disability Index (ODI).

3. Results

We examined 107 patients over 7 years to look at clinical and radiographic outcomes of MI-TLIF. A total of 66 females and 41 males were treated at our institution (average age 68.6, range 39–92). Levels fused included L1-L2 (n = 1, 1%), L2-L3 (n = 10, 9.3%), L3-L4 (n = 16, 15%), L4-L5 (n = 75, 70%), L5-S1 (n = 1, 1%), or multilevel fusion (n = 4, 3.7%). The average Cobb angle decreased from 21.6 ± 5.6 preoperatively to 15.63 ± 3.58 postoperatively ($p < 0.05$). The lumbar lordosis and pelvic incidence (PI-LL) mismatch was improved postoperatively (**Figure 1**). There were improvements in VAS (**Figure 2**), SF36 (**Figure 3**), and ODI (**Figure 4**). There was a statistically significant correlation between Cobb angle reduction and HRQOL

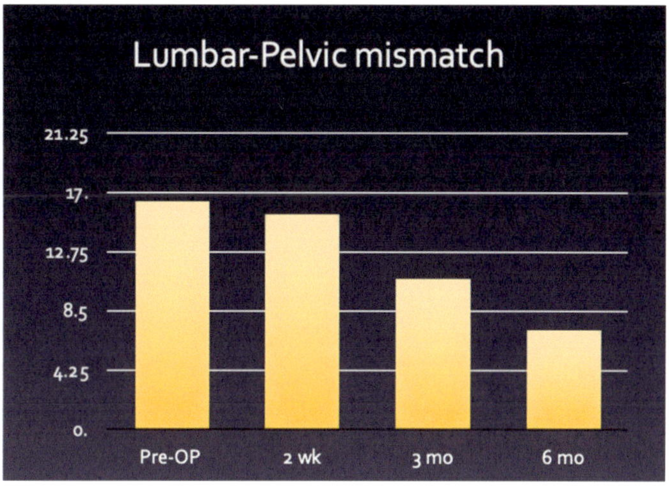

Figure 1.
Lumbar lordosis—pelvic incidence mismatch improved to <10 at 3 months postoperative period.

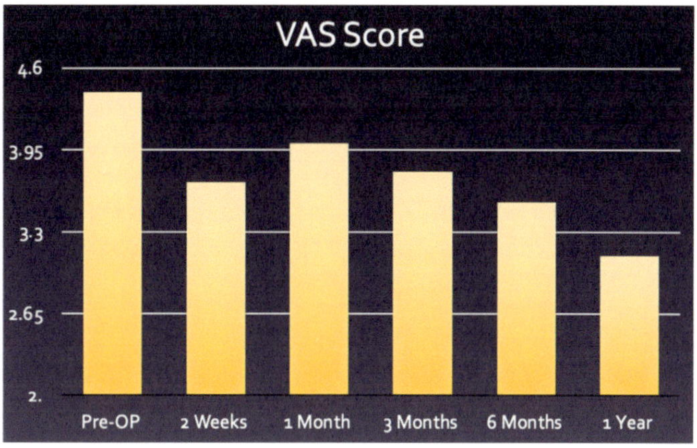

Figure 2.
Down trending of the VAS score from preoperative to 1 year postop.

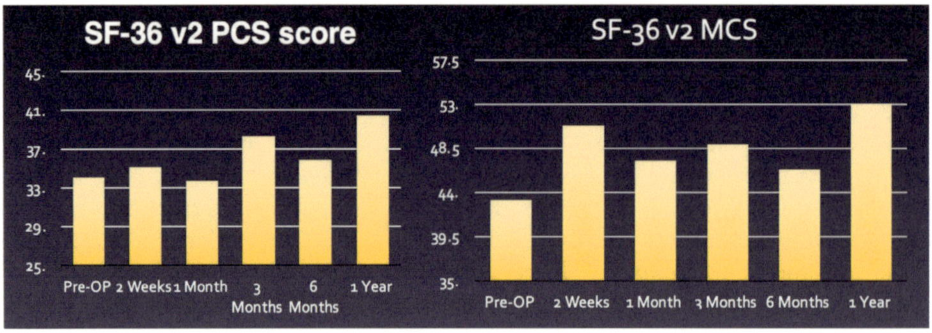

Figure 3.
Down trending of the SF36 PCS and MCS score from preoperative to 1 year postop.

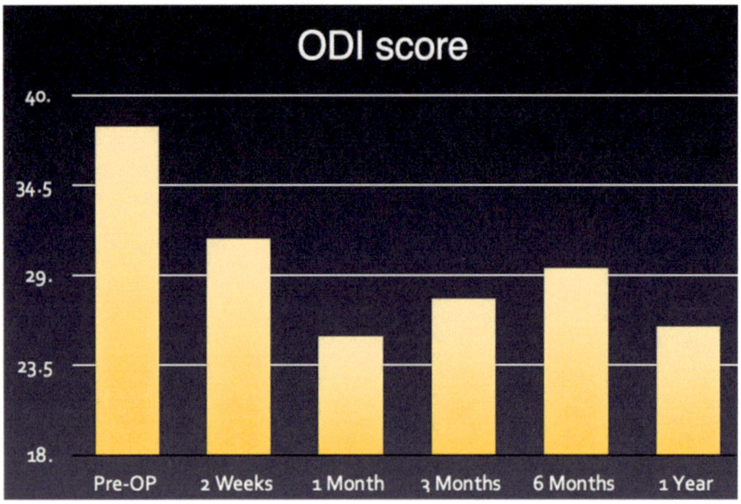

Figure 4.
Down trending of the ODI from preoperative to 1 year postop.

measure improvement ($p < 0.05$). Patients also exhibited an age-related trend, with average Cobb angles increasing with the patient's age. Cobb angles improved after MI-TLIF in 94% (n = 101) of patients and this improvement correlated with an improvement in symptom questionnaires. MI-TLIF resulted in a high rate of spinal fusion and a low rate of reoperation. Preoperative and intraoperative imaging of a patient who underwent an MI-TLIF procedure are demonstrated in **Figures** 5 and **6**. Cobb angles were reduced by 21% on average with just a single-level fusion, supporting the consideration of a focused single-level fusion versus a large multilevel fusion in cases of coronal deformity, especially in the elderly.

4. Discussion

Adult degenerative scoliosis (ADS) is recognized as the most common type of spinal deformity in skeletally mature individuals, which develops as a result of progressive and asymmetric degeneration of the vertebral column [12]. Back pain is

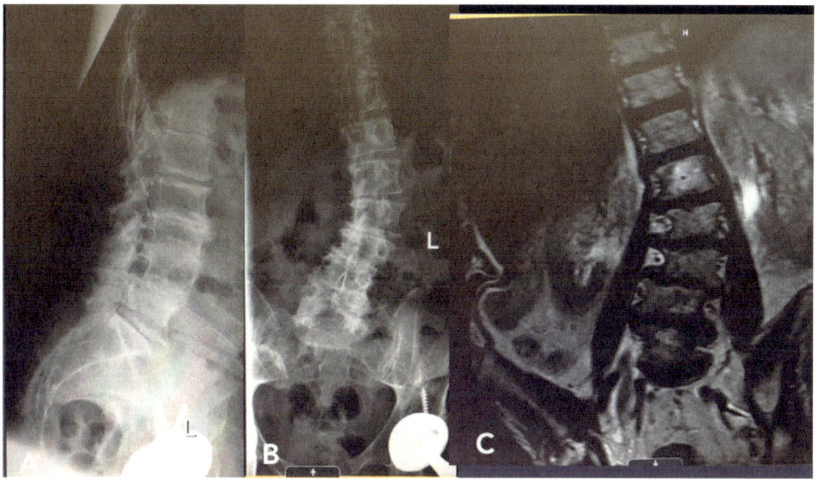

Figure 5.
Preoperative imaging of 72 year old female with symptomatic low back pain and neurogenic claudication. Neutral standing lateral (A) AP (B) plain radiographs and (C) MRI of the lumbosacral spine demonstrating coronal deformity of the lumbar spine.

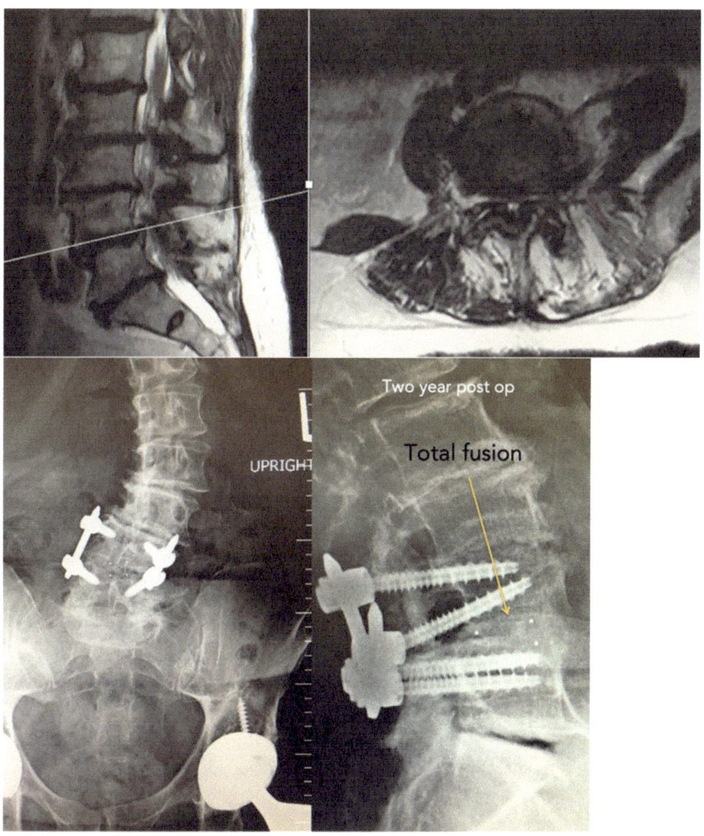

Figure 6.
MRI revealed most severe lumbar stenosis at L4–5, consistent with patient's distribution of radiculopathy. She then underwent focal treatment of the lumbar scoliosis with MIS TLIF L4–5. She experienced symptomatic relief and 2 year postop XR shows fusion at L4–5.

highly prevalent in adult scoliosis, it occurs most frequently on the convex aspect of the coronal deformity that is thought to be due to degenerative changes in intervertebral discs and facet joints, as well as para-spinal muscular exertion associated with spinal imbalance [10]. Debilitating radiculopathy has also been noted to occur in up to 78% of individuals suffering from ADS, which typically occurs on the concave side of the spinal deformity as a result of foraminal stenosis due to facet joint hypertrophy and lateral subluxation [13, 14]. Measurement of the Cobb angle is currently the gold standard for quantification of spinal curvature and is widely considered to be a reproducible technique for establishing the initial diagnosis of adult scoliosis, as well as a postoperative measurement of surgical success. The Cobb angle derives its name from John Robert Cobb, an American orthopedic surgeon, who pioneered the use of this measurement modality and described its use in his "Outline for the Study of Scoliosis" which was published as part of Instructional Course Lectures of the American Academy of Orthopedic Surgeons in 1948 [15]. In order to diagnose a skeletally mature individual with scoliosis, the Cobb angle, which is the resultant angle of intersecting perpendicular lines drawn parallel to the superior vertebral endplate of the most tilted vertebra at the top of the curve and the inferior endplate of the most titled vertebral body at the bottom of the curve, must be observed to be or exceed 10 degrees on a posteroanterior standing radiograph of the spine (**Figure** 7) [16]. Although it is important to radiographically assess the patient's spinal curvature prior to and after surgical intervention, it is equally important to assess other aspects that encompass the patient's well-being in order to obtain an accurate measure of surgical success.

Several outcomes are measured in order to assess the effect that scoliosis has on a patient's overall quality of life, as well as the clinical success of scoliosis repair surgery. Health-related Quality of Life (HRQOL) measures, such as Short Form-36 (SF-36), Visual Analog Scale (VAS), and Oswestry Disability Index (ODI) are the most frequently used measurement modalities. HRQOL explores physical, mental,

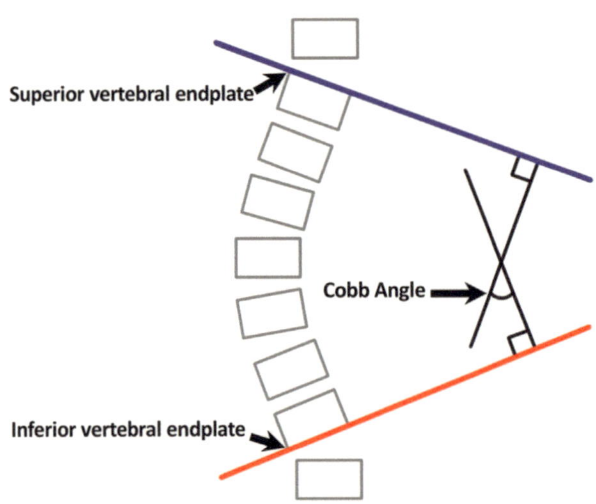

Figure 7.
Cobb angle. The resultant angle of intersecting perpendicular lines drawn parallel to the superior vertebral endplate of the most tilted vertebra at the top of the curve and the inferior endplate of the most titled vertebral body at the bottom of the curve, must be observed to be or exceed 10 degrees on a posteroanterior standing radiograph of the spine.

emotional, and even social parameters of a patient's subjective well-being. SF-36 is the most commonly used HRQOL that is composed of eight scale scores which include but are not limited to, physical functioning, bodily pain, general mental health, and social functioning, which yield physical component summary (PCS) and mental component summary (MCS) scores [17]. The VAS is frequently utilized to further assess a patient's degree and intensity of pain on a continuous scale that ranges from a score of 0 ("no pain") to 100 ("worst imaginable pain") [18]. The ODI is an equally important tool utilized in assessment of patients' ability to perform activities of daily living (ADL), lifting heavy objects, as well as other aspects of their lives that may be affected by spinal disorders. Furthermore, ODI can isolate the variable of physical impairment from its psychosocial consequences [19]. Once a patient is radiographically diagnosed with scoliosis, their symptoms severely affect their quality of life and are refractory to nonoperative methods of treatment, it may be time to consider surgical intervention. Decompression and instrumented fusion is frequently indicated in order to relieve neurogenic claudication and halt the devastating sequelae of curve progression, destabilization, and degeneration of vertebral bone architecture caused by adult degenerative scoliosis. Ever since the 1930s, when it was first reported in literature by Capener as a treatment for spondylolisthesis, lumbar spine fusion has been performed via anterior retroperitoneal approach, as it provides direct access to vertebral bodies and is associated with fusion rates of approximately 92% [20, 21]. However, anterior lumbar interbody fusion (ALIF) is not without complications as it carries an inherent risk of injury to various abdominal and retroperitoneal structures that include, but are not limited to, great vessels, abdominal organs, prevertebral ganglia, and plexus [22]. Although open spine surgery has been traditionally employed to gain access to lumbar spine and treat its associated deformities, minimally invasive approaches are now becoming commonplace due to their ability to significantly reduce surgical trauma, preserve paraspinal muscle, decrease intraoperative blood loss, and hospital stay [23]. Specifically, when comparing transforaminal lumbar interbody fusion (TLIF) to minimally invasive transforaminal lumbar interbody fusion (MI-TLIF), it is becoming more evident that the latter is superior in every aspect. Multiple investigations have established that MI-TLIF yields significantly better SF-36, VAS, and ODI scores, improved perioperative outcomes and long-term outcomes that are comparable to TLIF, as evidenced by multiple studies, including a four-year prospective investigation which revealed an overall bony fusion rate of 93.5% for MI-TLIF [24–26]. As supported by the aforementioned studies, it is clear that the minimally invasive approach is superior to that of the traditional open lumbar spine surgery, especially when considering the elderly patient population whose surgical outcomes are further complicated by comorbidities. Based on our results and the fact that minimally invasive spine surgery is associated with reduced intraoperative blood loss, it is indubitable that when compared to single-level, multilevel lumbar fusion results in a higher incidence of complications, especially in the elderly population [27].

4.1 Limitations

This study lacks a comparative arm in which patients underwent multilevel lumbar fusion for not only the fractional curve but also the major curve for similar presentations of predominant radiculopathy. We do not have such a comparison group due to the lack of aggressive surgeries for this particular patient population in our institution. Despite of that, this single-arm study is adequate to show the safety and long-term durability of single-level TLIF for patients with predominant radiculopathy from fractional curve.

5. Conclusions

There exists substantial evidence to support lumbar fusion procedures in cases of spondylolysis, spondylolisthesis, and other cases of sagittal deformity. However, coronal scoliotic deformity can also be a cause of low back and leg pain in a certain subset of patients. Single-level minimally invasive transforaminal lumbar interbody fusion yields significant reductions in coronal deformity, improvement in health-related quality of life measures, a high rate of spinal fusion, and a low rate of reoperation. This minimally invasive approach to the lumbar spine is especially important when considering single versus multilevel fusion for the treatment of adult degenerative scoliosis in the elderly patient population whose surgical outcomes are already at high risk due to comorbidities.

Author contributions

Conceptualization, N.H. and M.P.C.; methodology, N.H. and M.P.C.; formal analysis, N.H. and M.P.C.; investigation, N.H. and M.P.C.; resources, N.H. and M.P.C.; writing—original draft preparation, V.C., V.G. and T.M.E.; writing—review and editing, V.C., V.G., T.M.E., N.H. and M.P.C.; supervision, N.H. and M.P.C.; project administration, N.H. and M.P.C.

Funding

This research received no external funding.

Conflicts of interest

Mick Perez-Cruet MD, MS: Thompson MIS-ownership interest.

Author details

Mick Perez-Cruet* and Lee-Onn Chieng
Department of Neurosurgery, Corewell Health Beaumont University Hospital, USA

*Address all correspondence to: perezcruet@yahoo.com

References

[1] Smith JS, Shaffrey CI, Fu K-MG, Scheer JK, Bess S, Lafage V, et al. Clinical and radiographic evaluation of the adult spinal deformity patient. Neurosurgery Clinics of North America. 2013;**24**:143-156. DOI: 10.1016/j.nec.2012.12.009

[2] Hall JE. Spinal surgery before and after Paul Harrington. Spine. 1998;**23**:1356

[3] Dickson JH, Harrington PR. The evolution of the Harrington instrumentation technique in scoliosis. JBJS. 1973;**55**:993

[4] Liljenqvist U, Lepsien U, Hackenberg L, Niemeyer T, Halm H. Comparative analysis of pedicle screw and hook instrumentation in posterior correction and fusion of idiopathic thoracic scoliosis. European Spine Journal: Official Publication of the European Spine Society, the European Spinal Deformity Society, and the European Section of the Cervical Spine Research Society. 2002;**11**:336-343. DOI: 10.1007/s00586-002-0415-9

[5] Mohan AL, Das K. History of surgery for the correction of spinal deformity. Neurosurgical Focus. 2003;**14**:e1. DOI: 10.3171/foc.2003.14.1.2

[6] Youn MS, Shin JK, Goh TS, Kang SS, Jeon WK, Lee JS. Relationship between cervical sagittal alignment and health-related quality of life in adolescent idiopathic scoliosis. European Spine Journal. Oct 2016;**25**(10):3114-3119. DOI: 10.1007/s00586-016-4488-2 [Epub 2016 Mar 10]

[7] Smith JS, Lafage V, Shaffrey CI, Schwab F, Lafage R, Hostin R, et al. Outcomes of operative and nonoperative treatment for adult spinal deformity: A prospective, multicenter, propensity-matched cohort assessment with minimum 2-year follow-up. Neurosurgery. 2016;**78**:851-861. DOI: 10.1227/NEU.0000000000001116

[8] Glassman SD, Bridwell K, Dimar JR, Horton W, Berven S, Schwab F. The impact of positive sagittal balance in adult spinal deformity. Spine. 2005;**30**:2024-2029

[9] Roussouly P, Nnadi C. Sagittal plane deformity: An overview of interpretation and management. European Spine Journal. 2010;**19**:1824-1836. DOI: 10.1007/s00586-010-1476-9

[10] Birknes JK, White AP, Albert TJ, Shaffrey CI, Harrop JS. Adult degenerative scoliosis: A review. Neurosurgery. 2008;**63**:94-103. DOI: 10.1227/01.NEU.0000325485.49323.B2

[11] Hussain NS, Perez-Cruet MJ. Complication management with minimally invasive spine procedures. Neurosurgical Focus. 2011;**31**:E2. DOI: 10.3171/2011.8.FOCUS11165

[12] Schwab F, Dubey A, Gamez L, El Fegoun AB, Hwang K, Pagala M, et al. Adult scoliosis: Prevalence, SF-36, and nutritional parameters in an elderly volunteer population. Spine. 2005;**30**:1082-1085

[13] Graham RB, Sugrue PA, Koski TR. Adult degenerative scoliosis. Clinical Spine Surgery. 2016;**29**:95-107. DOI: 10.1097/BSD.0000000000000367

[14] Simmons ED. Surgical treatment of patients with lumbar spinal stenosis with associated scoliosis. Clinical Orthopaedics and Related Research. Mar 2001;(384):45-53

[15] Cobb JR. Outline for the study of scoliosis. In: Instructional Course

Lectures, the American Academy of Orthopaedic Surgeons. Vol. 5. Ann Arbor: J.W. Edwards; 1948. pp. 261-275

[16] Kane WJ. Scoliosis prevalence: A call for a statement of terms. Clinical Orthopaedics and Related Research. Jul-Aug 1977;(126):43-46. PMID: 598138

[17] Laucis NC, Hays RD, Bhattacharyya T. Scoring the SF-36 in orthopaedics: A brief guide. The Journal of Bone and Joint Surgery. American Volume. 2015;**97**:1628-1634. DOI: 10.2106/JBJS.O.00030

[18] Hawker GA, Mian S, Kendzerska T, French M. Measures of adult pain: Visual analog scale for pain (VAS pain), numeric rating scale for pain (NRS pain), McGill pain questionnaire (MPQ), short-form McGill pain questionnaire (SF-MPQ), chronic pain grade scale (CPGS), short form-36 bodily pain scale (SF-36 BPS), and measure of intermittent and constant osteoarthritis pain (ICOAP). Arthritis Care and Research. 2011;**63**(Suppl. 11):S240-S252. DOI: 10.1002/acr.20543

[19] Fairbank JCT, Pynsent PB. The oswestry disability index. Spine. 2000;**25**:2940

[20] Capener N. Spondylolisthesis. BJS. 1932;**19**:374-386. DOI: 10.1002/bjs.1800197505

[21] Saraph V, Lerch C, Walochnik N, Bach CM, Krismer M, Wimmer C. Comparison of conventional versus minimally invasive extraperitoneal approach for anterior lumbar interbody fusion. European Spine Journal. 2004;**13**:425-431. DOI: 10.1007/s00586-004-0722-4

[22] Samudrala S, Khoo LT, Rhim SC, Fessler RG. Complications during anterior surgery of the lumbar spine: An anatomically based study and review. Neurosurgical Focus. 1999;7:e9. DOI: 10.3171/foc.1999.7.6.10

[23] Mobbs RJ, Phan K, Malham G, Seex K, Rao PJ. Lumbar interbody fusion: Techniques, indications and comparison of interbody fusion options including PLIF, TLIF, MI-TLIF, OLIF/ATP, LLIF and ALIF. Journal of Spine Surgery. 2015;**1**:2-18. DOI: 10.3978/j.issn.2414-469X.2015.10.05

[24] Wong AP, Smith ZA, Stadler JA, Hu XY, Yan JZ, Li XF, et al. Minimally invasive transforaminal lumbar interbody fusion (MI-TLIF): Surgical technique, long-term 4-year prospective outcomes, and complications compared with an open TLIF cohort. Neurosurgery Clinics of North America. 2014;**25**:279-304. DOI: 10.1016/j.nec.2013.12.007

[25] Phan K, Huo YR, Hogan JA, Xu J, Dunn A, Cho SK, et al. Minimally invasive surgery in adult degenerative scoliosis: A systematic review and meta-analysis of decompression, anterior/lateral and posterior lumbar approaches. Journal of Spine Surgery. 2016;**2**:89-104. DOI: 10.21037/jss.2016.06.07

[26] Perez-Cruet MJ, Hussain NS, White GZ, Begun EM, Collins RA, Fahim DK, et al. Quality-of-life outcomes with minimally invasive transforaminal lumbar interbody fusion based on long-term analysis of 304 consecutive patients. Spine. 2014;**39**:E191-E198. DOI: 10.1097/BRS.0000000000000078

[27] Mahesh B, Upendra B, Vijay S, Kumar GA, Reddy S. Complication rate during multilevel lumbar fusion in patients above 60 years. Indian Journal of Orthopaedics. 2017;**51**:139-146. DOI: 10.4103/0019-5413.201704

Chapter 2

Minimally Invasive Approaches to Adult Spinal Deformity Correction

Rouzbeh Motiei-Langroudi, Saeed Abdollahifard and Uduak-Obong I. Ekanem

Abstract

The management of adult spinal deformity has undergone a transformative shift with the emergence of minimally invasive approaches. Traditionally, the correction of complex spinal curvatures necessitated extensive open surgeries to perform the osteotomies and instrumentation, contributing to long and high-risk operations. However, the advent of minimally invasive techniques has ushered in a new era of patient-centric care. These innovative approaches entail smaller incisions, reduced tissue disruption, and advanced navigational tools that in many instances yield satisfactory and comparable results. The benefits are manifold: decreased blood loss, shorter hospitalizations, faster recovery times, and improved patient satisfaction. This chapter highlights the profound impact of these techniques on patient outcomes and healthcare systems. Nonetheless, challenges remain. Surgeons must navigate a steep learning curve, and there are limitations in addressing severe deformities through minimally invasive means. Rigorous patient selection and meticulous preoperative planning are pivotal to achieving success.

Keywords: minimally invasive, surgery, spine, deformity, adult

1. Introduction

Adult spinal deformity (ASD) is a spectrum of diseases involving both lumbar and thoracic regions and consisting of adult degenerative scoliosis, degenerative sagittal plane deformities, and iatrogenic spinal deformities [1, 2]. Given that number of geriatric patients over 65 in the United States is expected to double by 2050 compared to 2010, and there is evidence that shows the overall prevalence of ASD in older patients is close to 68%, proper attention and appropriate interventions should be taken into account before it causes major burdens and disabilities to the patients [3, 4]. Based on the severity of the disease, patients may experience a spectrum of symptoms such as axial or radicular pain, claudication, walking disturbance, and symptoms of spinal stenosis [2, 5, 6]. Different treatment options are available for patients with ASD. Conservative therapy, including physical therapy, medications, and a combination of interventional pain procedures has been the first line of treatment [7–9]. Surgery could be reserved for those refractories to conservative management and those with worsening deformity, significant neurological deficits and symptoms disrupting patients' activities of daily living [4, 10–12]. Open techniques to correct the deformity have been in practice for decades with good results; however, there is a growing body of evidence and interest in the minimally invasive surgery (MIS) techniques nowadays [13]. In a study by Lak et al., a review of 350 cases of adult degenerative scoliosis revealed that open surgery and MIS showed comparable improvement in outcomes of patients. However, better outcome was associated with open surgery and better safety outcomes with MIS [14]. Another study by Dangelmajer et al. reported no significant difference in the complication rates between the open surgical approach and MIS [15]. Current evidence could not draw a solid conclusion regarding the superiority of MIS vs. open surgery techniques, and recent studies emphasize individualized surgical planning for each patient [16]. In this chapter, we will delve into the application of MIS for ASD, patient selection (i.e., an algorithm to decide which patients are a better fit for MIS or hybrid vs. open), advantages and disadvantages of MIS vs. open techniques, different MIS techniques, and possible future advances.

2. Definitions

Before proceeding, some definitions and indexes should be reviewed.

2.1 Coronal cobb angle (CCA)

The angle between two lines perpendicular to the lines extending from the superior (cephalic spine body) and inferior (caudal) endplates of the most tilted spine vertebral bodies [17].

2.2 Pelvic incidence-lumbar lordosis (PI-LL) mismatch

Pelvic incidence (PI) is defined as an angle between a line drawn from the middle of the head of the femoral bone to the midpoint of sacrum superior endplate and a line perpendicular to the middle of the sacral endplate [18]. Lumbar lordosis (LL) is traditionally determined by the Cobb angle between the upper endplates of the first lumbar (L1) and either the lower endplate of L5 or the upper endplate of S1 [19]. The discrepancy between PI and LL, referred to as PI-LL mismatch or discordance, is correlated with the patient's quality of life (QoL), and a mismatch of more than 10 degrees suggests misalignment as it is an indicator of maladaptation of the lumbar region to the pelvic anatomy [20].

2.3 Sagittal vertical Axis (SVA)

The term SVA refers to the measurement of the horizontal distance between two points on lateral full-body standing X-rays. C7-S1 SVA refers to the distance between the posterior superior part of S1 endplate and a plumb line drawn from the center of C7 [21], assessing in accordance with the upper thoracic to the pelvis. To take neck posture into account, C2 and Cranial Center of Gravity (CCoG) SVAs are proposed, measuring the distance between the posterior superior part of S1 endplate and a plumb line passing through the middle of C2 vertebral body and external auditory meatus, respectively [20]. It has been found that these indexes are associated with pain and QoL of patients [22].

2.4 Coronal vertical Axis (CVA)

Similar to SVA, CVA is measured on an anterior-posterior full-body standing X-rays. The most commonly used is C7-S1 CVA, as the distance measured between the midpoint of S1 endplate and a vertical plumb line passing through the midpoint of C7 vertebral body.

2.5 Pelvic tilt (PT)

PT is an angle between a vertical line drawn from the center of the head of the femoral bone and another line from the head of the femoral bone to the middle part of the superior endplate of S1. This term refers to the orientation of the pelvis in relation to the femoral head. Like previous measurements, it is correlated with the QoL and health condition of patients [20, 23].

Of note, these are only a few of several other measurements related to surgical planning for ASD patients. Readers are referred to other chapters or references for a full review of these.

3. Background, emergence, and development of MIS techniques

While initially developed and implemented in the 1990s to perform thoracic and lumbar discectomy and laminectomy in limited series [24, 25], the development of tubular retraction systems advanced the field of minimally invasive spine surgery [26, 27]. As MIS became more popular, conventional fusion techniques were implemented in MIS, initially including pedicle screw fusion (MIS-PSF), Transforaminal Lumbar Interbody Fusion (MIS-TLIF), and Posterior Lumbar Interbody Fusion (MIS-PLIF) [28–30]. Overall, these techniques were associated with decreased blood loss and pain and accelerated recovery time [31–33]. Later, newer MIS techniques were developed for fusion, such as Anterior Lumbar Interbody Fusion (ALIF), trans-psoas Lateral Lumbar Interbody Fusion (MIS-LLIF/TP), anterior-to-psoas Oblique Lumbar Interbody Fusion (MIS-OLIF/ATP), and trans-Kambin Oblique Lateral Lumbar Interbody Fusion (MIS-OLLIF) [34, 35]. Overall, these new approaches let surgeons access the spinal bodies from various angles [36].

With the development of advanced fusion techniques, MIS has been routinely implemented in deformity correction, either as MIS-alone techniques or combined with open techniques (hybrid approaches). To gain better global sagittal balance, Anterior Column Release (ACR) is added to anterolateral approaches. The goal is to release the anterior longitudinal ligament (ALL) and place a hyperlordotic interbody cage, to gain more sagittal correction. Currently, there is a growing trend toward less invasive procedures, and MIS techniques for ASD are rapidly progressing. These techniques are trying to achieve a higher success rate, fewer adverse events, faster recovery times, and provide better correction and alignment rates.

4. Overview of MIS techniques for ASD correction

4.1 Interbody fusion techniques

The utilization of interbody devices stands as a pivotal component within the realm of MIS deformity correction. In this context, the benefits extend beyond the fundamental aspects of load sharing and the enhancement of fusion rates—rationales commonly associated with their application in spinal surgery at large. As executing multi-level and higher-grade osteotomies through MIS means remains the main challenge, thereby a significant portion of the curve correction should be obtained through interbody devices. Consequently, the meticulous selection of the appropriate interbody technique stands as a pivotal cornerstone of surgical planning.

Various factors play a role in the choice of interbody fusion route: 1) past surgical history (spine, abdominal, and vascular): anterolateral approaches are riskier in those with multiple abdominal and vascular surgeries; 2) degree of correction needed: better sagittal and coronal correction obtained through anterolateral approaches; 3) need for direct decompression (as opposed to indirect decompression only): generally needed for those with severe canal stenoses, direct decompression is better achieved through posterior approaches; and 4) higher body mass indexes (generally more than 35–37) make anterolateral approaches less doable.

4.1.1 Posterior interbody fusion techniques

Including two techniques (PLIF and TLIF), their main advantages include: single approach surgery (i.e., no need to reposition), ability to be performed at any lumbosacral level, absence of anatomical restrictions, and providing direct decompression (added to indirect). However, their biggest disadvantage of MIS deformity surgery is that they provide less restoration of lumbar lordosis per level, compared to anterolateral approaches. Moreover, their ability to correct coronal curves is very limited, making them a less suitable option for these curves. With the advent of expandable devices, there are some hopes to provide better sagittal correction, but their use so far has been limited mostly to short-segment fusions and has not been an integral part of deformity correction. Lastly, their smaller size provides a smaller device-endplate contact surface area, making proper deformity correction less achievable.

4.1.2 Anterolateral interbody fusion techniques

One of the first non-posterior interbody approaches devised, ALIF, might not conventionally be considered MIS by all. However, advent of newer retracting systems, avoidance of cutting posterior lumbar muscles, and retroperitoneal trajectories, make it an ideal MIS technique. Primarily used at L5-S1 and L4-L5, it has a wider range of available lordotic and hyper-lordotic options, making it a strong tool for the restoration of segmental lordosis and sagittal balance. Also, it is more efficient in providing coronal restoration than the posterior options. ALIF also allows for resection of ALL and sometimes posterior longitudinal ligament (PLL), adding to its deformity correction potential. The inclusive disadvantage of the technique is a risk of vascular injuries and safe access being limited to L4-S1.

LLIF/TP can be safely performed in most upper and mid-lumbar levels (L1-L2 to L2-L4), but also at L4-L5, though with some difficulty due to the anatomy of iliac crest. Availability of a wide range of lordotic and hyper-lordotic options, providing a large device-endplate contact surface area, and adding bilateral endplate coverage to the benefits, it is a strong option for sagittal correction and by far the strongest interbody option to restore coronal curves. The main disadvantage is, however, the risk of direct or more commonly retraction injury to lumbar plexus nerves [37, 38].

The anatomic limitations of ALIF and LLIF/TP, paved the way for the advent of OLIF/ATP approach [39]. Always a left-sided approach which uses the corridor between psoas muscle and aorta/left common iliac artery at L1-L5 and the corridor between right and left common iliac arteries (like ALIF) at L5-S1, it has a lower risk of lumbar plexus injury compared to LLIF and lower risk of vascular injury compared to ALIF (although more than LLIF) [38, 40]. In terms of deformity correction, they are strong tools in both sagittal and coronal curve correction (comparable to LLIF). Moreover, their anatomic approach makes ALL release more accessible than LLIF, adding to the benefit.

Regardless of the choice, all MIS interbody options are valuable integral parts of MIS deformity correction. A meta-analysis of a total of 18 studies and 732 ASD patients undergoing deformity correction showed that all-posterior MIS options were associated with shorter operative times compared to lateral. MIS lateral options (LLIF and OLIF) were superior to MIS and open posterior options in terms of blood loss and length of hospital stay. Both MIS options resulted in similar fusion rates, and functional and radiological outcomes, compared to open [41].

4.2 Anterior column release techniques

Although MIS is reported to be effective in improving the global sagittal and coronal alignment, its efficacy is less than open techniques for the correction of severe imbalances, especially if only relies on interbody devices to correct the deformity [42]. These limitations led to the development of new techniques, including Anterior Column Release (ACR) [43]. Mostly done as a part of a lateral trans-psoas or oblique anterior-to-psoas approach to perform complete discectomy and release of the ALL, followed by placement of a hyper-lordotic (20–30°) interbody device, ACR enables surgeons to achieve similar effectiveness as open surgery through an MIS approach [42, 44]. The primary reports showed promising effects, although these results were limited by the small sample size of studies [45].

As ACR is relatively new, long-term data on its complication profile and efficacy is still missing. However, early data exploring the efficiency of ACR performed as a part of LLIP/TP has been very promising, and 20–30° of sagittal correction, 10–15° of coronal correction, and 5–10° of PT correction has been achieved through ACR alone. More importantly, the complications are less, especially in terms of blood loss (average ~ 50 mL) compared to open osteotomy techniques including pedicle subtraction osteotomy (PSO) and vertebral column resection (VCR), which are traditionally associated with a substantial blood loss (occasionally even up to 1–2 L). All these earlier results have been achieved through a combination of LLIF/TP and ACR. However, ACR is achievable through an OLIF/ATP (and potentially ALIF), as both approaches provide excellent access to ALL. The main complication after ACR, like other anterolateral approaches, has been reported to be anterior thigh weakness and numbness, which in most cases fully resolves within 1–2 years after surgery. This complication can be further reduced and avoided with various modifications, including minimization of retraction time, limiting the exposure, employment of neuromonitoring, flexing hips and knees, and not breaking the surgical table [46–49]. In general, ACR has been reported to obtain similar radiographic results compared to open osteotomy counterparts, with significantly less estimated blood loss and similar overall complication rates.

4.3 Osteotomy techniques

The current use of posterior osteotomy techniques during MIS approaches is limited to "mini-open" posterior column osteotomies (PCOs) and PSOs, which are obtained through smaller-than-open incisions, periosteal dissection only at the level of osteotomies, followed by the closure of the osteotomies across the percutaneous pedicle screws and the connecting rods through a cantilever force [34, 50]. As technically not different from the open or mini-open osteotomies, these are better addressed in other chapters, but their knowledge is necessary for spine surgeons to increase the amount of correction obtained via MIS and hybrid approaches.

4.4 Posterior fusion techniques

All previously mentioned techniques should be complemented by posterior fusion. Pedicle and iliac screws are placed in a percutaneous technique in the desired levels, either spanning from the upper (mostly T3-T5) or lower (usually T9-T11) thoracic to sacropelvic region, followed by advancing two rods under the fascia to connect the screws. No different than other MIS pedicle screw placement techniques else than the number of levels included in the fusion, details of these techniques are addressed elsewhere.

4.5 Bone graft techniques

Special attention should be paid for bone graft options during MIS surgery. As MIS surgery classically does not expose posterolateral bone, the template and basis for bony fusion are significantly limited in these surgeries. Moreover, relying more on instrumentation for deformity correction and decompression provides less autograft, compared to open counterparts. As such, surgeons need to have a good knowledge base of various bone graft options and surgical techniques that improve bony fusion. These include proper preparation of endplates during interbody device placement to maximize device-endplate interaction, use of larger interbody devices (through anterolateral approaches) if possible, maximizing the number of interbodies used, harvesting as much autograft as possible (plus considering harvesting more from remote sites), and finally proper use of allografts to include all stages and properties needed for new bone formations (osteogenesis, osteo-induction, and osteo-conduction).

5. Advantages and disadvantages of MIS for patients with ASD

Due to the less invasive nature of MIS techniques, these procedures are intriguing for both surgeons and patients. The main advantages of MIS are decreased tissue dissection and disruption and, as a result, less muscle atrophy, lower risk of infection and blood loss, shorter length of hospital stay, and faster recovery of patients [13, 34, 51, 52]. Nevertheless, some points should be considered before choosing MIS techniques to treat patients with ASD. In addition to having a steeper learning curve, both surgical staff and patients may be exposed to a greater amount of radiation [53–55]. Additionally, MIS surgery may have limited effectiveness in correcting severe deformities, which makes it less suitable for such cases. However, newer techniques are being developed to address this issue [14].

5.1 Efficacy

Acknowledging the promising nature of MIS in addressing ASD, still the biggest question is how it compares with open approaches in terms of clinical and radiographic outcomes. A systematic review and meta-analysis by Lak et al. in 2020 included four retrospective cohorts and 350 patients to compare the efficacy of open surgery vs. MIS for patients with ASD. Although the results were inconsistent among studies, open surgery resulted in a greater change of SVA and PI-LL mismatch. Regarding the change in the leg and back pain and disability, overall, there was a significant decrease in back pain, leg pain, and disability in both MIS and open surgery groups without a significant difference between the two groups [14]. Mittal et al. conducted a systematic review and meta-analysis (2023) of the outcomes of patients following open and MIS surgeries in patients with ASD. This review included 18 studies and 732 patients and divided studies into the subgroup of lateral approaches (LLIF and OLIF) and posterior approaches (PLIF and TLIF). The latter subgroup was subdivided into MIS and open surgery further. The results of meta-analyses showed that both lateral and posterior groups could significantly reduce leg pain, back pain, disability of patients (measured by Oswestry Disability Index or ODI), Cobb angle, and SVA. It is worth mentioning that the difference between lateral and posterior subgroups was not significant in the above-mentioned analyses. In terms of the total operation time, the pooled time for the lateral approach was 401 minutes (only one study), while it was 233 minutes for MIS posterior (four studies) and 380 for open posterior (four studies) approaches; the difference was not significant between posterior approaches. Five studies in the lateral approach reported only interbody fusion time, resulting in a pooled operation time of 170 minutes. The fusion rate was determined to be 97.8% (four studies) and 96.6% (six studies) in the lateral and posterior groups, respectively; these differences were not statistically significant either. Length of hospital stay was shortest in the lateral group (with a pooled rate of 4.15 days across four studies) and the longest in the posterior open surgery (13.54 days across four studies), and the difference between these groups was significant. The posterior MIS group had a pooled rate of 6.25 days across two studies. The result might indicate overall faster recovery in the MIS approach compared to open surgery. Moreover, the study investigated the complications in addition to efficacy. According to the results, lower blood loss was achieved by the posterior MIS approach compared to the open posterior approach (385 mL vs. 1325 mL, respectively). One study in the lateral group reported total blood loss (477 mL), and three others reported blood loss only during fusion (86 mL). The difference in blood loss between the lateral and open posterior approaches was found to be significant. No significant difference was noted for other complications such as durotomy, permanent neurologic and device-related adverse events, re-operation rate, and pseudoarthrosis between MIS and open approaches [41]. In a study on ASD patients in whom three-column osteotomy was not performed, post-operative ODI, Scoliosis Research Society (SRS) score, and European Quality of life (EQ-5D) scores were all comparable between circumferential MIS (cMIS) and open patients. Both versions were also equally effective in correcting CCA, PI-LL mismatch, SVA, and PT. Confirming other results, open patients had more blood loss and shorter operative times, compared with cMIS patients. Interestingly, revision rates were similar between the two groups. Of note, excluding 3-level osteotomy cases from the study leaves severe deformity cases out, considering open surgery might be more efficient in correcting severe curves [56]. Lastly, another study comparing the complication rates of open, hybrid, and MIS techniques (among

60 patients) concluded that although there was no difference in the rate of overall complications, a significantly lower rate of intraoperative complications was observed in the MIS [13]. Added to the efficacy of MIS techniques in improving clinical outcomes, global sagittal and coronal parameters, and spinopelvic parameters, they have been shown to improve fractional curves as well, resulting in clinical improvement in radiculopathy symptoms. In a study on patients with fractional curves worse than 10 degrees undergoing either open or cMIS surgeries, both groups had comparable reductions in fractional curves and leg pain after surgery [57].

Combining the benefits of both MIS (less tissue disruption, minimal blood loss, faster recovery, etc.) and open (more efficiency and greater curve correction) surgeries, hybrid procedures seem to be interesting and now widely used alternatives. In a study, hybrid procedures were shown to correct CCA better than cMIS, while they both yielded comparable results in the correction of SVA, PI-LL mismatch, PT, and sacral slope (SS). At 2 years, cMIS had better ODI scores and a greater ODI change compared to baseline, less back pain and greater VAS back pain change, compared to hybrid techniques. All these outcomes were comparable at 3 years mark between cMIS and hybrid, except leg pain, which was lower for cMIS compared to hybrid. cMIS had fewer complications overall compared to hybrid techniques, except for pseudarthrosis (i.e., higher rate in cMIS) [58].

Nonetheless, not all studies have shown comparable results for MIS vs. open. Uribe et al. conducted a multicenter study to compare the outcomes and complications of patients with ASD who underwent open, MIS, and hybrid surgery in a propensity-matched cohort, each group consisting of 20 patients. Investigating radiographic outcomes, their results showed that open and hybrid approaches were superior to MIS in terms of improving PI-LL mismatch, thoracic CCA, thoracic kyphosis, and C7-S1 SVA. However, all 3 versions were successful in improving lumbar CCA. Comparing the clinical outcomes, all these procedures could decrease back pain (using a visual analog scale (VAS)) and disability (ODI) of patients, but the results for reducing leg pain were again superior to open surgery. The hybrid surgery had the longest overall operation time, while the open surgery had the shortest time. However, the length of hospitalization was the opposite, with patients who underwent hybrid surgery staying for a shorter period compared to others [13].

As evident in these results, studies are not consistent in terms of imaging and radiographic outcomes. However, most studies conclude that at least for less severe and moderate deformities, MIS approaches are associated with comparable outcomes to open surgery. In severe cases, it can be concluded that open approaches obtain superior results. However, almost all studies agree upon the fact that MIS is associated with less blood loss, shorter hospital stays, and faster recovery.

MIS may provide additional promising outcomes in terms of proximal junction kyphosis (PJK). PJK is radiologically defined as a Cobb angle of more than 20 degrees or an increase of more than 10 degrees postoperatively cranial to the site of surgery between the upper instrumented vertebra (UIV) and the vertebra 2 levels rostral to UIV (UIV + 2). In general, 39% of patients who undergo surgery for correction of spine deformity may be affected, but not all patients will be symptomatic [59, 60]. Gandhi et al. found that the incidence of PJK after surgery for ASD was lower for MIS versions (ACR and LLIF) compared to open surgery [61].

5.2 Costs

A retrospective cohort of 71 patients tried to evaluate the costs of MIS for adult degenerative scoliosis and compare it to the open technique. This study concluded that the total inpatient charges were significantly lower for the MIS group ($269 K vs. $391 K), while there were no significant differences in terms of the need for inpatient rehabilitation after hospitalization [62]. Another study by Swamy et al. compared the cost-effectiveness of MIS (12 patients) and open surgery (10 patients) for patients with adult degenerative scoliosis. This cohort reported fewer total costs for the MIS group ($83 K vs. $111 K, adjusted to Canadian dollars), while open surgery costs less in uncomplicated cases ($47 K vs. $76 K). Also, it has been reported that MIS is associated with higher quality-adjusted life years leading to the conclusion that MIS is less expensive than the open approach [63]. Chung et al. conducted a review study and confirmed previous findings on the economic aspects of spine surgery techniques, including both MIS and open surgery, without limiting the analysis to the ASD [64].

6. Case selection

With the new advancements in MIS techniques and the lack of clear superiority of one technique over the other, now surgeons (and patients) have more tools in their armamentarium to tackle this challenging disease. Instead of choosing one over the other, there have been some efforts to recommend a tailored and case-by-case approach. Despite the controversies, most authors believe that the applicability of MIS is more limited in the case of a severe sagittal imbalance or in patients with prior fusions. Although recent advances such as ACR and mini-PSO have been used to address the limitation of MIS for severe deformities in addition to keeping the minimally invasive advantages, open surgery with osteotomy might still be the preferred option in revision surgeries in patients with severe deformities [44]. Mummaneni et al. developed an MIS deformity surgery algorithm (MISDEF) to help physicians to decide whether to proceed with MIS or open surgery [65]. In this algorithm, three classes of treatments, including MIS decompression with or without fusion, decompression with interbody fusion, and open surgery with osteotomy and fusion up to the thoracic region, were introduced regardless of the health condition or age of the patients. This algorithm was revised in 2018 to include ACR, mini-open PSO, expandable cages, and hybrid techniques. In general, for non-fused or flexible spines, SVA less than 6 cm, PT < 25, PI-LL mismatch less than 10 degrees, and CCA less than 20 degrees, MIS with decompression or combined with a fusion at the listhetic level was recommended, leaving the more severe cases amenable to open surgery [34, 66].

However, more advancements have been made since the publication of these algorithms and comfort level of spine surgeons with MIS techniques has increased, making them able to handle more severe cases with MIS surgeries. More importantly, patients' comorbidities, past surgical history (specifically abdominal and spine), and body status favor one choice over the other. In our opinion, patients needing higher degrees of sagittal curve correction (more than 50–55 degrees), fusions anticipated to go to upper thoracic, those with previous spine surgeries resulting in multi-level and long-segment fusions, history of complex abdominal and vascular surgeries, those with multi-level severe central stenosis (needing direct multi-level decompression), and those with less optimal body status (BMI > 35–37) are a better fit for open techniques. On the other hand, those with coronal-dominant curves, severe coronal imbalance, sagittal correction needs below 50–55, lack of previous spine surgeries or short-segment fusions at most, and those with a more favorable BMI are perfect fits for MIS. In patients with coronal imbalance, it is worth mentioning that the type of curve has a significant role in outcome after MIS correction, and as a result choice of

MIS vs. open. Those with a balanced (less than 3 cm) C7-S1 CVA (type A) and those with a coronal malalignment (C7-S1 CVA > 3 cm) shifted toward concavity of the main lumbar curve (type B) can be successfully handled through an MIS approach. Those with a coronal malalignment shifted toward convexity of the main lumbar curve (type C) are prone to worsened coronal imbalance after addressing the fractional lumbar curve, and as such are not ideal candidates for MIS [67]. As previously noted, above and beyond all, the surgeon's expertise and comfort level with either technique is perhaps the most critical factor in the choice of surgery.

7. Conclusions

The current era is exciting with the wealth and plethora of surgical options to address ASD. In the absence of a clear benefit of one technique over the other in most patients, modern-day surgeons and clinicians should be well aware and trained by MIS as well as open techniques to tailor their proposed treatment to patients' needs.

Author details

Rouzbeh Motiei-Langroudi[1*], Saeed Abdollahifard[1,2] and Uduak-Obong I. Ekanem[3]

1 Department of Neurosurgery, University of Kentucky, Lexington, KY, USA

2 Research Center for Neuromodulation and Pain, Shiraz, Iran

3 School of Medicine, Tulane University School of Medicine, New Orleans, LA, USA

*Address all correspondence to: rouzbeh.motiei@uky.edu

References

[1] Kim HJ, Yang JH, Chang D-G, Lenke LG, Suh SW, Nam Y, et al. Adult spinal deformity: A comprehensive review of current advances and future directions. Asian Spine Journal. 2022;**16**(5):776-788

[2] Kim HJ, Yang JH, Chang DG, Suk SI, Suh SW, Song KS, et al. Adult spinal deformity: Current concepts and decision-making strategies for management. Asian Spine Journal. 2020;**14**(6):886-897

[3] Schwab F, Dubey A, Gamez L, El Fegoun AB, Hwang K, Pagala M, et al. Adult scoliosis: Prevalence, SF-36, and nutritional parameters in an elderly volunteer population. Spine. 2005;**30**(9):1082-1085

[4] Ames CP, Scheer JK, Lafage V, Smith JS, Bess S, Berven SH, et al. Adult spinal deformity: Epidemiology, health impact, evaluation, and management. Spine Deformity. 2016;**4**(4):310-322

[5] Smith JS, Fu K-M, Urban P, Shaffrey CI. Neurological symptoms and deficits in adults with scoliosis who present to a surgical clinic: Incidence and association with the choice of operative versus nonoperative management. Journal of Neurosurgery: Spine. 2008;**9**(4):326-331

[6] de Kleuver M, Faraj SSA, Haanstra TM, Wright AK, Polly DW, van Hooff ML, et al. The Scoliosis Research Society adult spinal deformity standard outcome set. Spine Deformity. 2021;**9**(5):1211-1221

[7] Everett CR, Patel RK. A systematic literature review of nonsurgical treatment in adult scoliosis. Spine. 2007;**32**(19):S130-S1S4

[8] Glassman SD, Berven S, Kostuik J, Dimar JR, Horton WC, Bridwell K. Nonsurgical resource utilization in adult spinal deformity. Spine. 2006;**31**(8):941-947

[9] Youssef J, Orndorff D, Patty C, Scott M, Price H, Hamlin L, et al. Current status of adult spinal deformity. Global Spine Journal. 2013;**3**(1):051-062

[10] Fu K-MG, Bess S, Shaffrey CI, Smith JS, Lafage V, Schwab F, et al. Patients with adult spinal deformity treated operatively report greater baseline pain and disability than patients treated nonoperatively; however, deformities differ between age groups. Spine. 2014;**39**(17):1401-1407

[11] Fu K-MG, Smith JS, Sansur CA, Shaffrey CI. Standardized measures of health status and disability and the decision to pursue operative treatment in elderly patients with degenerative scoliosis. Neurosurgery. 2010;**66**(1):42-47

[12] Glassman SD, Schwab FJ, Bridwell KH, Ondra SL, Berven S, Lenke LG. The selection of operative versus nonoperative treatment in patients with adult scoliosis. Spine. 2007;**32**(1):93-97

[13] Uribe JS, Deukmedjian AR, Mummaneni PV, Fu K-MG, Mundis GM, Okonkwo DO, et al. Complications in adult spinal deformity surgery: An analysis of minimally invasive, hybrid, and open surgical techniques. Neurosurgical Focus. 2014;**36**(5):E15

[14] Lak AM, Lamba N, Pompilus F, Yunusa I, King A, Sultan I, et al. Minimally invasive versus open surgery for the correction of adult

degenerative scoliosis: A systematic review. Neurosurgical Review. 2021;**44**(2):659-668

[15] Dangelmajer S, Zadnik PL, Rodriguez ST, Gokaslan ZL, Sciubba DM. Minimally invasive spine surgery for adult degenerative lumbar scoliosis. Neurosurgical Focus FOC. 2014;**36**(5):E7

[16] Deukmedjian AR, Ahmadian A, Bach K, Zouzias A, Uribe JS. Minimally invasive lateral approach for adult degenerative scoliosis: Lessons learned. Neurosurgical Focus FOC. 2013;**35**(2):E4

[17] Oakley PA, Ehsani NN, Harrison DE. The scoliosis quandary: Are radiation exposures from repeated X-rays harmful? Dose Response. 2019;**17**(2):1559325819852810

[18] Chen H-F, Zhao C-Q. Pelvic incidence variation among individuals: Functional influence versus genetic determinism. Journal of Orthopaedic Surgery and Research. 2018;**13**(1):59

[19] Iyer S, Sheha E, Fu MC, Varghese J, Cunningham ME, Albert TJ, et al. Sagittal spinal alignment in adult spinal deformity: An overview of current concepts and a critical analysis review. JBJS Reviews. 2018;**6**(5):e2

[20] Savarese LG, Menezes-Reis R, Bonugli GP, Herrero C, Defino HLA, Nogueira-Barbosa MH. Spinopelvic sagittal balance: What does the radiologist need to know? Radiologia Brasileira. 2020;**53**(3):175-184

[21] Katzman WB, Parimi N, Gladin A, Fan B, Wong SS, Mergenthaler J, et al. Reliability of sagittal vertical axis measurement and association with measures of age-related hyperkyphosis. Journal of Physical Therapy Science. 2018;**30**(12):1417-1423

[22] Glassman SD, Bridwell K, Dimar JR, Horton W, Berven S, Schwab F. The impact of positive sagittal balance in adult spinal deformity. Spine (Phila Pa 1976). 2005;**30**(18):2024-2029

[23] Lafage V, Schwab F, Patel A, Hawkinson N, Farcy JP. Pelvic tilt and truncal inclination: Two key radiographic parameters in the setting of adults with spinal deformity. Spine (Phila Pa 1976). 2009;**34**(17):E599-E606

[24] Obenchain TG. Laparoscopic lumbar discectomy: case report. Journal of Laparoendoscopic Surgery. 1991;**1**(3):145-149

[25] Horowitz MB, Moossy JJ, Julian T, Ferson PF, Huneke K. Thoracic discectomy using video assisted thoracoscopy. Spine (Phila Pa 1976). 1994;**19**(9):1082-1086

[26] Foley KT. Microendoscopic discectomy. Techniques in Neurosurgery. 1997;**3**:301-307

[27] Schick U, Döhnert J, Richter A, König A, Vitzthum HE. Microendoscopic lumbar discectomy versus open surgery: An intraoperative EMG study. European Spine Journal. 2002;**11**(1):20-26

[28] Briggs H, Milligan PR. Chip fusion of the low back following exploration of the spinal canal. JBJS. 1944;**26**(1):125-130

[29] Harms J, Rolinger H. A one-stager procedure in operative treatment of spondylolistheses: Dorsal traction-reposition and anterior fusion (author's transl). Zeitschrift fur Orthopadie und ihre Grenzgebiete. 1982;**120**(3):343-347

[30] Foley KT. Advances in minimally invasive spine surgery. Clinical Neurosurgery. 2002;**49**:499-517

[31] Villavicencio AT, Burneikiene S, Roeca CM, Nelson EL, Mason A.

Minimally invasive versus open transforaminal lumbar interbody fusion. Surgical Neurology International. 2010;**1**:12

[32] Momin AA, Steinmetz MP. Evolution of minimally invasive lumbar spine surgery. World Neurosurgery. 2020;**140**:622-626

[33] Prabhu MC, Jacob KC, Patel MR, Pawlowski H, Vanjani NN, Singh K. History and evolution of the minimally invasive Transforaminal lumbar Interbody fusion. Neurospine. 2022;**19**(3):479-491

[34] Lovecchio F, Qureshi SA. The current state of minimally invasive approaches to adult spinal deformity. Current Reviews in Musculoskeletal Medicine. 2019;**12**(3):318-327

[35] Ozgur BM, Aryan HE, Pimenta L, Taylor WR. Extreme lateral Interbody fusion (XLIF): A novel surgical technique for anterior lumbar interbody fusion. The Spine Journal. 2006;**6**(4):435-443

[36] Pawar A, Hughes A, Girardi F, Sama A, Lebl D, Cammisa F. Lateral lumbar Interbody fusion. Asian Spine Journal. 2015;**9**(6):978-983

[37] Spitnale MJ, Thier ZT, Grabowski G. Lateral lumbar Interbody fusion at the L5-S1 vertebral level: A unique anatomical case report. Cureus. 2022;**14**(2):e22096

[38] Xu DS, Walker CT, Godzik J, Turner JD, Smith W, Uribe JS. Minimally invasive anterior, lateral, and oblique lumbar interbody fusion: A literature review. Annals of Translational Medicine. 2018;**6**(6):104

[39] Silvestre C, Mac-Thiong JM, Hilmi R, Roussouly P. Complications and morbidities of mini-open anterior retroperitoneal lumbar Interbody fusion: Oblique lumbar Interbody fusion in 179 patients. Asian Spine Journal. 2012;**6**(2):89-97

[40] Woods K, Fonseca A, Miller LE. Two-year outcomes from a single Surgeon's learning curve experience of oblique lateral Interbody fusion without intraoperative Neuromonitoring. Cureus. 2017;**9**(12):e1980

[41] Mittal S, Sudhakar PV, Ahuja K, Ifthekar S, Yadav G, Sinha S, et al. Deformity correction with Interbody fusion using lateral versus posterior approach in adult degenerative scoliosis: A systematic review and observational meta-analysis. Asian Spine Journal. 2023;**17**(2):431-451

[42] Godzik J, Pereira BA, Hemphill C, Walker CT, Wewel JT, Turner JD, et al. Minimally invasive anterior longitudinal ligament release for anterior column realignment. Global Spine Journal. 2020;**10**(2 Suppl):101s-110s

[43] Saigal RAB, Eastlack RK, Bagheri A, Tran S, Brown D, et al. Anterior column realignment: Analysis of neurological risk and radiographic outcomes. Neurosurgery. 2020;**87**(3):E347-EE54

[44] Januszewski J, Vivas AC, Uribe JS. Limitations and complications of minimally invasive spinal surgery in adult deformity. Annals of Translational Medicine. 2018;**6**(6):109

[45] Cheung ZB, Chen DH, White SJW, Kim JS, Cho SK. Anterior column realignment in adult spinal deformity: A case report and review of the literature. World Neurosurgery. 2019;**123**:e379-ee86

[46] Murray GBJ, Bach K, Smith DA, Dakwar E, Uribe JS. Complications and neurological deficits following minimally

invasive anterior column release for adult spinal deformity: A retrospective study. European Spine Journal. 2015;**24**:397-404

[47] Saigal RAB, Eastlack RK, Bagheri A, Tran S, Brown D, Bagheri R, et al. Anterior column realignment: Analysis of neurological risk and radiographic outcomes. Neurosurgery. 2020;**87**(3):e347-e354

[48] Xu ZLF, Chen G, Chen Q. Reassessment system and staged surgical strategy with minimally invasive techniques for treatment of severe adult spinal deformities. World Neurosurgery. 2019;**126**:e860-e8e8

[49] Mundis GM TJ Jr, Kabirian N, Pawelek J, Eastlack RK, Uribe J, Klineberg E, et al. Anterior column realignment has similar results to pedicle subtraction osteotomy in treating adults with sagittal plane deformity. World Neurosurgery. 2017;**105**:249-256

[50] Wang MY, Bordon G. Mini-open pedicle subtraction osteotomy as a treatment for severe adult spinal deformities: Case series with initial clinical and radiographic outcomes. Journal of Neurosurgery: Spine. 2016;**24**(5):769-776

[51] Fan S, Hu Z, Zhao F, Zhao X, Huang Y, Fang X. Multifidus muscle changes and clinical effects of one-level posterior lumbar interbody fusion: Minimally invasive procedure versus conventional open approach. European Spine Journal. 2010;**19**(2):316-324

[52] Patel AA, Zfass-Mendez M, Lebwohl NH, Wang MY, Green BA, Levi AD, et al. Minimally invasive versus open lumbar fusion: A comparison of blood loss, surgical complications, and hospital course. The Iowa Orthopaedic Journal. 2015;**35**:130-134

[53] Kim CH, Lee CH, Kim KP. How high are radiation-related risks in minimally invasive Transforaminal lumbar Interbody fusion compared with traditional open surgery?: A meta-analysis and dose estimates of ionizing radiation. Clinical Spine Surgery. 2016;**29**(2):52-59

[54] Mariscalco MW, Yamashita T, Steinmetz MP, Krishnaney AA, Lieberman IH, Mroz TE. Radiation exposure to the surgeon during open lumbar microdiscectomy and minimally invasive microdiscectomy: A prospective, controlled trial. Spine (Phila Pa 1976). 2011;**36**(3):255-260

[55] Patel PD, Canseco JA, Houlihan N, Gabay A, Grasso G, Vaccaro AR. Overview of minimally invasive spine surgery. World Neurosurgery. 2020;**142**:43-56

[56] LV C, D, Chan AY, Passias P, Mundis GM, Eastlack RK, Fu KM, et al. Patient outcomes after circumferential minimally invasive surgery compared with those of open correction for adult spinal deformity: Initial analysis of prospectively collected data. Journal of Neurosurgery Spine. 2021;**36**(2):1-12

[57] MP CD, Anand N, Nunley P, La Marca F, Fu KM, Fessler R, et al. Treatment of the fractional curve of adult scoliosis with circumferential minimally invasive surgery versus traditional, open surgery: An analysis of surgical outcomes. Global Spine Journal. 2018;**8**(8):827-833

[58] ER CAK, Fessler RG, Than KD, Chou D, Fu KM, Park P, et al. Two- and three-year outcomes of minimally invasive and hybrid correction of adult spinal deformity. Journal of neurosurgery. Spine. 2021;**36**(4):595-608

[59] Mendoza-Lattes S, Ries Z, Gao Y, Weinstein SL. Proximal junctional kyphosis in adult reconstructive spine surgery results from incomplete restoration of the lumbar lordosis relative to the magnitude of the thoracic kyphosis. The Iowa Orthopaedic Journal. 2011;**31**:199-206

[60] Dubousset J, Diebo BG. Proximal junctional kyphosis in modern spine surgery: Why is it so common? Spine Surgery and Related Research. 2023;**7**(2):120-128

[61] Gandhi SV, Januszewski J, Bach K, Graham R, Vivas AC, Paluzzi J, et al. Development of proximal junctional kyphosis after minimally invasive lateral anterior column realignment for adult spinal deformity. Neurosurgery. 2019;**84**(2):442-450

[62] Uddin OM, Haque R, Sugrue PA, Ahmed YM, El Ahmadieh TY, Press JM, et al. Cost minimization in treatment of adult degenerative scoliosis. Journal of Neurosurgery. Spine. 2015;**23**(6):798-806

[63] Swamy G, Lopatina E, Thomas KC, Marshall DA, Johal HS. The cost effectiveness of minimally invasive spine surgery in the treatment of adult degenerative scoliosis: A comparison of transpsoas and open techniques. The Spine Journal. 2019;**19**(2):339-348

[64] Chung AS, Ballatori A, Ortega B, Min E, Formanek B, Liu J, et al. Is less really more? Economic evaluation of minimally invasive surgery. Global. The Spine Journal. 2021;**11**(1_suppl):30s-36s

[65] Mummaneni PV, Shaffrey CI, Lenke LG, Park P, Wang MY, La Marca F, et al. The minimally invasive spinal deformity surgery algorithm: A reproducible rational framework for decision making in minimally invasive spinal deformity surgery. Neurosurgical Focus. 2014;**36**(5):E6

[66] Choy W, Miller CA, Chan AK, Fu KM, Park P, Mummaneni PV. Evolution of the minimally invasive spinal deformity surgery algorithm: An evidence-based approach to surgical strategies for deformity correction. Neurosurgery Clinics of North America. 2018;**29**(3):399-406

[67] Walker CTGJ, Angel S, Giraldo JP, Turner JD, Uribe JS. Coronal balance with circumferential minimally invasive spinal deformity surgery for the treatment of degenerative scoliosis: Are we leaning in the right direction? Journal of Neurosurgery Spine. 2021;**34**(6):879-887

Chapter 3

Perspective Chapter: Sacral Alar Iliac Screws

Pablo Pazmiño

Abstract

Often during the reconstruction of Adult and Pediatric Spinal Deformities pedicle screw fixation is insufficient and a distal anchor with pelvic fixation is of paramount importance. Various techniques regarding the methodologies of Spinopelvic fixation (SPF) and placement of Sacral-1 Alar Iliac (S1AI) and Sacral-2 Alar Iliac (S2AI) screws has been described in the literature. While there is some consensus among the various techniques and angles utilized, these are often difficult to reproduce in an operative setting. Recently navigation systems have allowed for the successful navigation of the Sacro Alar Iliac corridor without screw complications, however not every facility has this technology on hand. Therefore, proficiency with the safe and accurate placement of Sacroalar iliac (SAI) screws using standard fluoroscopic imaging becomes a vital technique when circumstances demand ample distal fixation. To our knowledge, a definitive step by step review of the sacroalar iliac technique warrants description in order to delineate the insertion point and exact fluoroscopic imaging which can help confirm the safe placement of SAI screws through the anatomical corridor.

Keywords: Sacral-1 Alar Iliac Screws (S1AI), Sacral-2 Alar Iliac (S2AI) screws, scoliosis, lumbar degenerative disc disease, lumbar disc herniation, herniated disc, Sacroalar iliac (SAI) screws

1. Introduction

During revision surgery or reconstructive procedures spine surgeons are confronted with the need for sufficient distal spinopelvic fixation. There are several conventional approaches towards addressing sacro-pelvic fixation, each facing distinct challenges in the operative setting. Often in order to perform sacroalar iliac (SAI) screw fixation there are certain factors which must be taken into consideration. Careful deliberation over the exact number of SAI screws needed for the construct should be contemplated. Bone density and the pullout strength of any prior hardware needs to be taken into account. Screw prominence also plays a role and must be considered when evaluating patients' body habitus and relevant soft tissue coverage [1, 2]. Imaging and hospital equipment needs to be planned well in advance if computer navigation or robotic instrumentation needs to be accounted for. The goal of this chapter is to introduce the relevant anatomical entry points, bony morphology and fluoroscopic imaging required to safely place Sacral Alar Iliac Screws in the bony anatomic corridor in efforts towards achieving sufficient distal fixation for all spinal constructs.

 IntechOpen

2. Surgical technique and pearls

2.1 Positioning

The patient is positioned prone on a radiolucent table and all bony prominences are padded. The following anatomical landmarks should be palpated, marked, and recognized: The anterior inferior iliac spine (AIIS), posterosuperior iliac spine (PSIS), the posteriorinferior iliac spine (PIIS), the median sacral crest, the lateral sacral crest and the greater trochanter. Initially the base of the fluoroscopic image intensifier should be positioned on the opposite side of the table as the surgeon. The midline is marked and the area should be prepped and draped in standard fashion with careful placement of the drapes as distally as possible along the intergluteal cleft.

2.2 Bony anatomy and morphology

Morphologically the entry point for the SAI screws lies near the intersection of the lateral sacral crest and a line drawn midway between the outermost lateral rim of the S1 and S2 dorsal sacral foramina (**Figure 1**). A distinct osseous landmark is often difficult to visualize attributing to the overhang from the PSIS and the upward slope of the lateral sacral crest. Dissection near the lateral sacral crest may stir up bleeding from the foraminal arterial branches of the lateral sacral artery. There will also be filiform nerve fibers from the dorsal branches of the sacral nerves [3]. The literature describes a wide range of specific insertion points and trajectories for the SAI screws which can be difficult to reproduce in the operative theater [3–5]. In light of this the following technique uses fluoroscopic imaging to help confirm the safe placement of SAI screws in vivo.

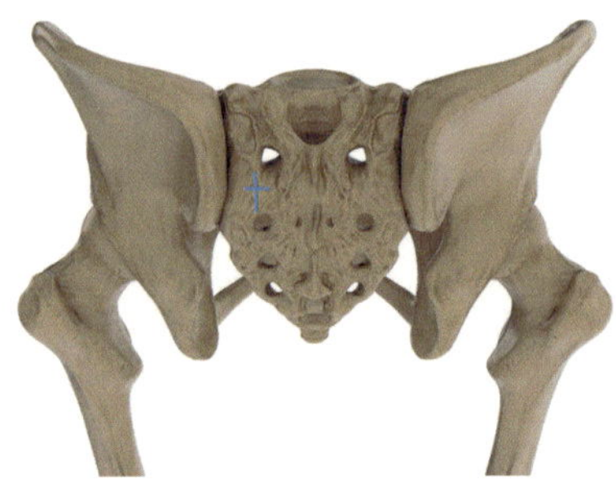

Figure 1.
Entry point for SAI screws lies near the intersection of the lateral sacral crest and a line drawn midway between the outermost lateral rim of the S1 and S2 dorsal sacral foramina.

2.3 Instrumentation and implants

An oscillating drill with a 3.5 mm threaded guide wire or a curved awl is used to cross the sacroiliac joint and along its course will ultimately penetrate the two cortices of the sacrum and the outer iliac cortex in a trajectory towards the anterior inferior iliac spine (**Figure 2A** and **B**). For ease of ultimate screw placement a long threaded guidewire can be inserted and then confirmed radiographically. If the imaging demonstrates a trajectory that is not ideal in any plane, a second guidewire can be situated next to the initial trajectory in order to provide any needed course correction, then the first guidewire can be removed (**Figures 3** and **4**). Consideration at this

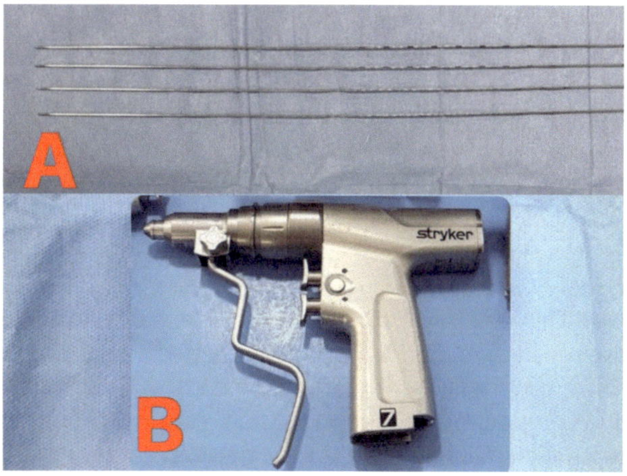

Figure 2.
(A) 3.5 mm Threaded guide wires, (B) Oscillating drill.

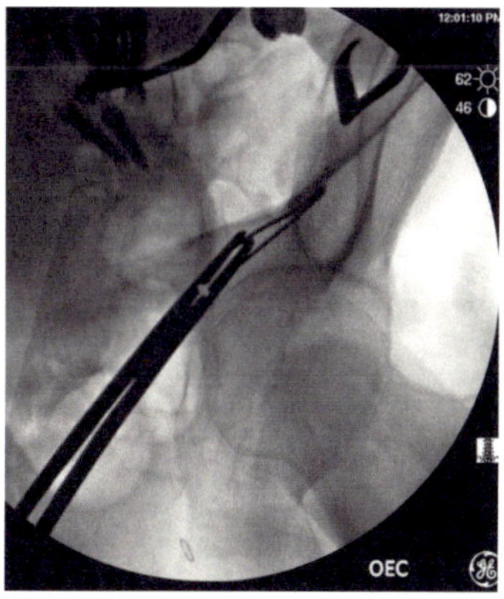

Figure 3.
In order to achieve optimal placement a second guidewire can be inserted in a different plane from the initial guide wire.

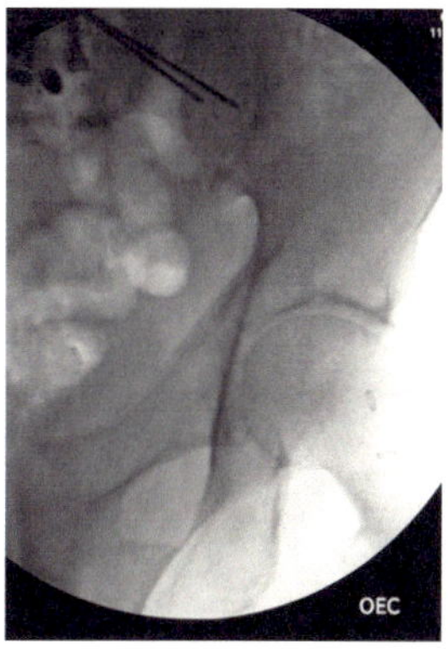

Figure 4.
Each guide wire can be visualized fluoroscopically, then the optimal trajectory can be selected based on fluoroscopic imaging. Once proper trajectory has been confirmed the second guidewire can be removed with the oscillating drill.

point should be made if there are one or two SAI screws being placed in order to allow sufficient clearance as the trajectories are being set and defined.

3. Fluoroscopic imaging

3.1 Entry point

The obturator outlet view (OOV) renders an inclined teardrop outline along the involved hemipelvis. This teardrop structure itself represents the superimposition of anterior and posterior columns. This bony teardrop reflects the sacroiliac osseous corridor wherein the SAI screw will reside (**Figures** 5 and **6**). The tubular shaped corridor resembles the geometric configuration of a frustrum (**Figure** 7). In order to obtain a proper OOV/teardrop view starting from a neutral Anteroposterior (AP) position, the fluoroscopic intensifier should be angled approximately 20–30° cephalad in the coronal plane, and then rotated over the involved hemipelvis 20–30° until the widest possible teardrop can be visualized while leaving a sufficient rim of the anterior inferior iliac

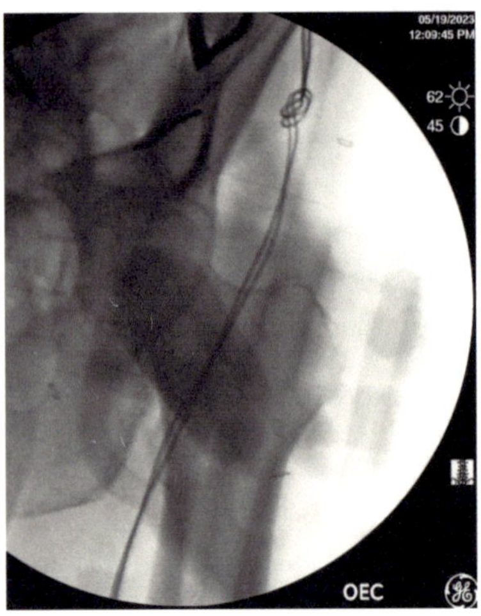

Figure 5.
Fluoroscopy view demonstrating the bony teardrop along the sacroiliac osseous corrido, with the tip of the guidewire in the northern corner of the teardrop.

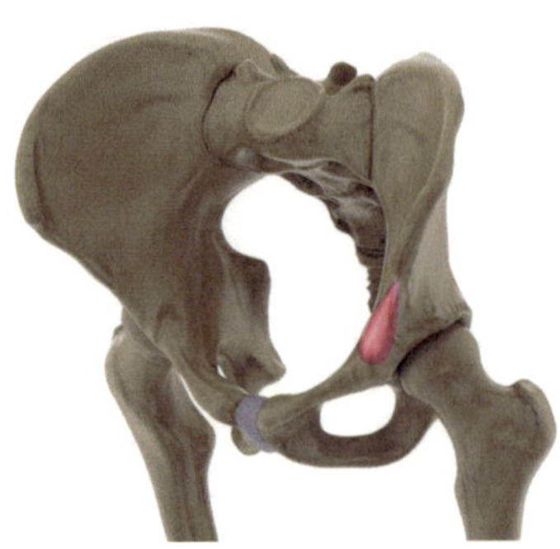

Figure 6.
Animation reflecting the bony teardrop visualized during the obturator outlet view.

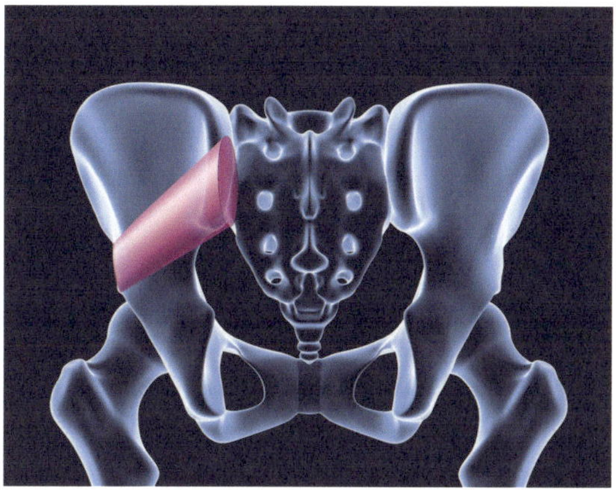

Figure 7.
In geometry a frustrum is the three dimensional shaped object enclosed between the two planes of another solid, it is similar to a cone with the pointed tip of the cone removed. This pink tubular shaped bony corridor represents the channel through which the SAI screws must traverse.

spine's outer ridge (**Figures 8–10**). On the fluroscopy view optimal placement of the teardrop should sit above the femoral head and the acetabular sulcus (**Figures 5** and **10**).

Once the entry point has been established, another threaded guide wire can be placed parallel to the first wire in order to accommodate two screws in the SAI corridor. Alternatively, if the construct necessitates only a single screw then at this point the threaded guide wire can be advanced to assure positioning over the sciatic notch and within the margins of the iliac wing. Ideal placement within the teardrop for a single screw has been found to be at the intersection of lines formed by the longest possible horizontal/transverse line which can be drawn along the width of the teardrop, and a vertical line dropped from the apex of the teardrop itself [6]. Final correct placement of the screw should demonstrate the entire screw lies securely within the confines of the bony teardrop which represents the frustrum spanning the entire bony sacroalar iliac corridor (**Figures 11–14**).

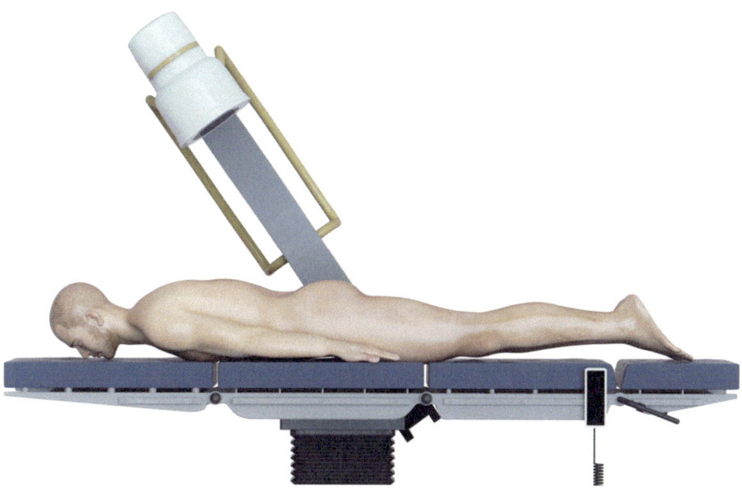

Figure 8.
Step 1: In order to obtain the obturator teardrop view (OOV), first the fluoroscopic intensifier should be angled approximately 20–30° cephalad in the coronal plane.

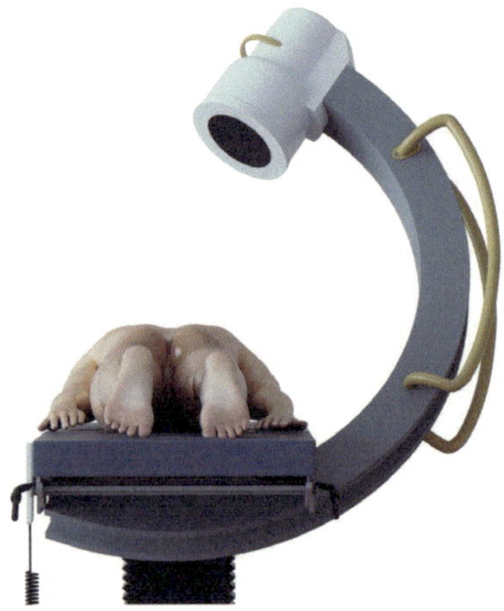

Figure 9.
Step2: Next the intensifier should be rotated over the involved hemipelvis another 20–30° until the widest possible teardrop can be visualized while leaving a sufficient rim of the anterior inferior iliac spine's outer ridge.

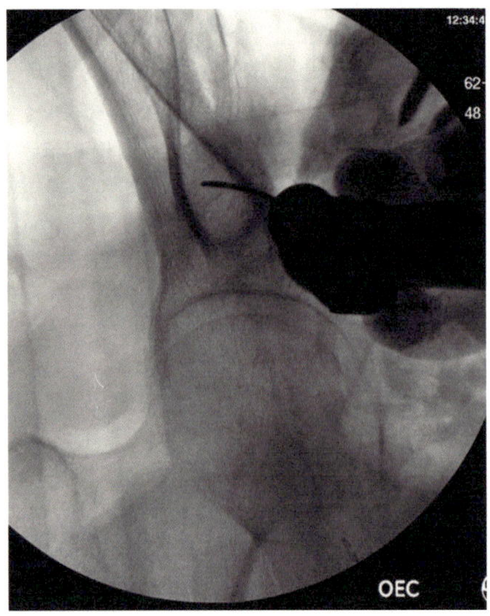

Figure 10.
Step3: Rotate the Carm over the involved hemipelvis until a distinct teardrop is visualized while also leaving a sufficient lateral rim of the anterior inferior iliac spine. Final placement should center the teardrop over the femoral head and acetabular sulcus.

3.2 Advancement

In order to confirm safe advancement within the frustrum sequential radiographic views must be obtained. First a standard AP View can be utilized to help identify the S1 Endplate, the S1 and S2 Foramen. While in this position a manual palpation of the bony prominences of the Anterior Inferior Iliac Spine (AIIS) and the greater trochanter can serve as relevant landmarks for screw trajectory. The guide wire can be meticulously advanced on the AP view to check the cranio caudal angle as the pin needs to pass 35 mm inside sacral bone and then within the ilium it would need to traverse another 35–65 mm of cancellous bone [3].

The next imaging that should be obtained is an inlet and outlet view which can confirm accurate placement within the sciatic buttress and corroborate that no medial violation has occurred towards the neurovascular structures and/or bladder (**Figures 11–14**).

As a final view a true lateral image should be obtained where both sciatic notches are perfectly superimposed (**Figure 15**). This will serve as the primary view for guidewire insertion and screw final advancement. On the lateral image great care should be taken to identify the acetabulum and the greater Sciatic Notch, while ensuring the wire is headed towards the AIIS. Ideally the shaft of the screw should reside

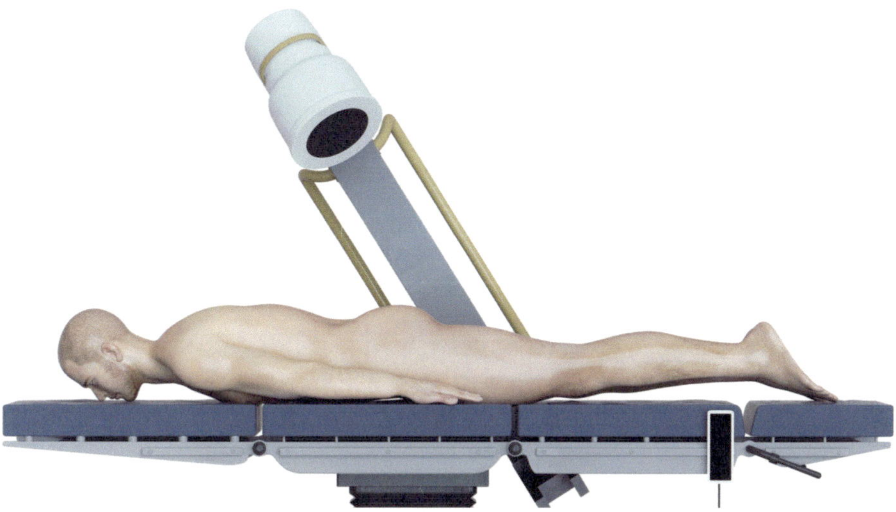

Figure 11.
Inlet view: This caudad projection of the pelvic bony rim is obtained by tilting the fluoroscopy 35–45° cephalad.

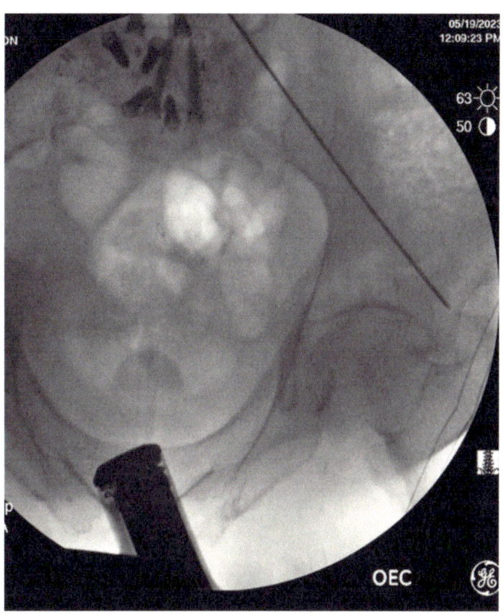

Figure 12.
Inlet view demonstrating the threaded guidewire within the bony confines of the sacroalar iliac corridor. On this view ensure the guide wire has not violated the pelvic rim medially.

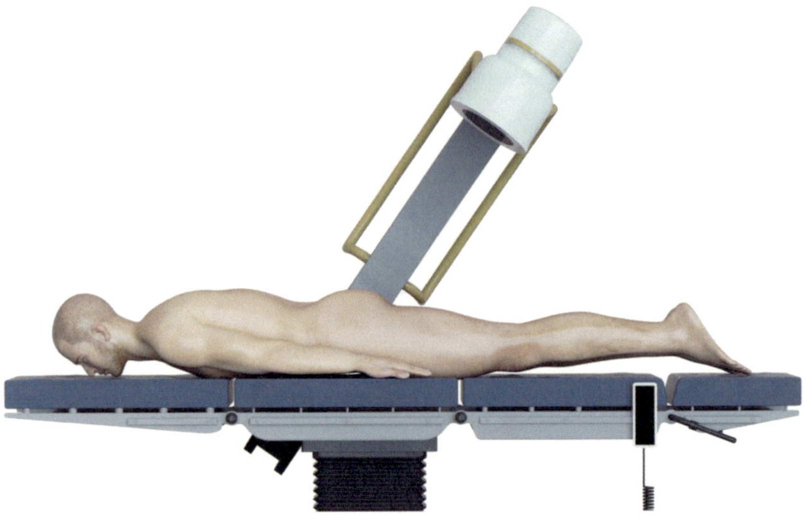

Figure 13.
Outlet view: This cephalad projection is perpendicular to the plane of the sacrum and is obtained by aiming the C-arm 35–45° caudad.

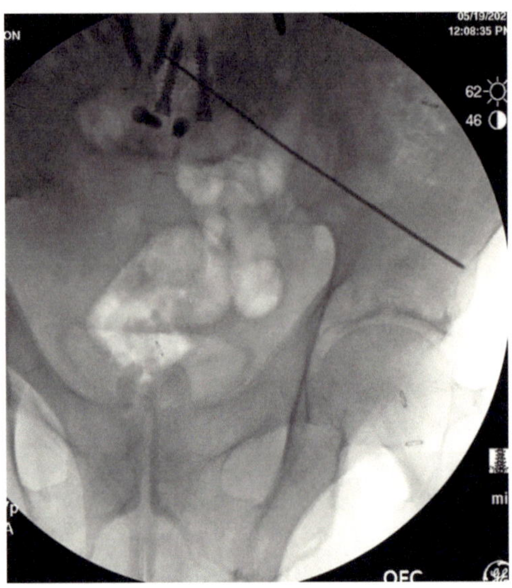

Figure 14.
This outlet view provides further confirmation the threaded guidewire is within the bony constraints of the sciatic buttress and pelvis.

1–2 cm above the acetabulum and the threads of the screw should graze the cortico-cancellous junction of the bone adjacent to the sciatic notch.

3.3 Screw placement

The cannulated screw itself can be placed in line with the threaded guidewire and advanced under fluoroscopy. The guidewire can be removed and visualized on fluoroscopy, prior to final screw placement. Alternatively, if an awl is used then it can

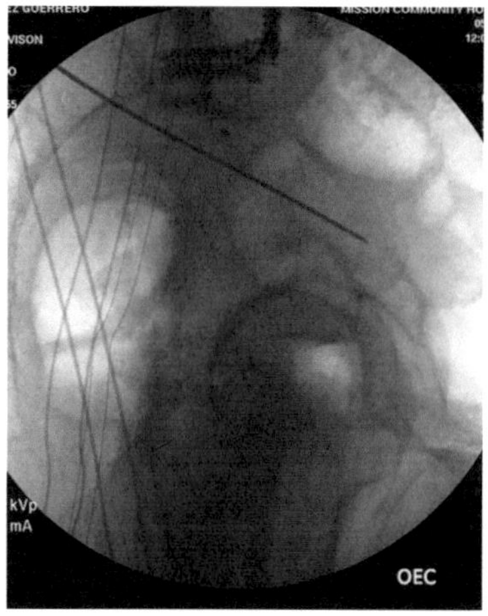

Figure 15.
On a true lateral view confirmation of proper guidewire placement above the acetabulum and sciatic notch can be confirmed.

be removed and the path can be palpated with a ball probe prior to screw placement. Final screw dimensions are typically a width either 8–9 mm and a length ranging from 70 to 110 mm [3]. Prior to final screw placement a 6 or 7 mm tap can be inserted under fluoroscopic visualization. Final screw positioning can be confirmed on the Iliac Oblique View which provides a lengthwise lateral view of the entire screw to reconfirm placement above the acetabulum and sciatic notch.

3.4 Case study

61 year old male presents with intense lumbar complaints which are 50% bilateral leg pain and 50% low back pain. The radiculopathy in the legs were rated 6–8 out of ten. The radicular pains were more severe in the right leg. The patient has tried and failed a course of conservative measures inclusive of transforaminal epidural

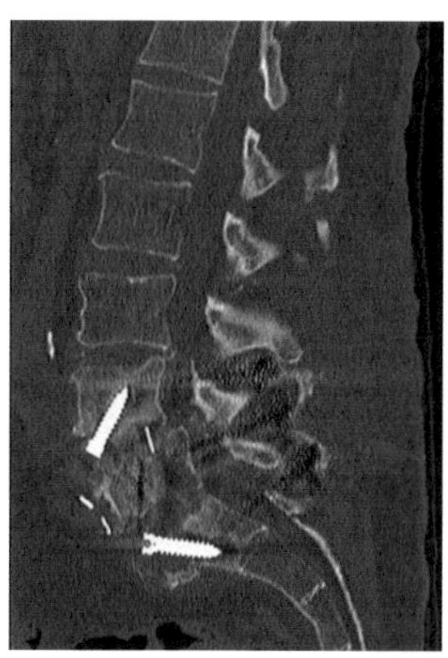

Figure 16.
Lumbar CT Sagittal 3month postoperative views demonstrating significant hardware lucency and the need for hardware revision with sacroiliac alar screws in order to achieve distal fixation.

injections, physical therapy, bracing, acupuncture, and Nonsteroidal anti inflammatories. Lumbar MRI and CT scans demonstrated a considerable amount of hardware loosening, and significant lucency around the hardware (**Figures 16** and **17**). The decision was made to remove the prior hardware, secure proximal fixation, and obtain distal Sacral alar-iliac hardware fixation (**Figures 18** and **19**). Postoperatively the patient noted a resolution of both back pain and radiculopathy and returned to regular activities including work within three months. He remained asymptomatic at his one year postoperative appointment.

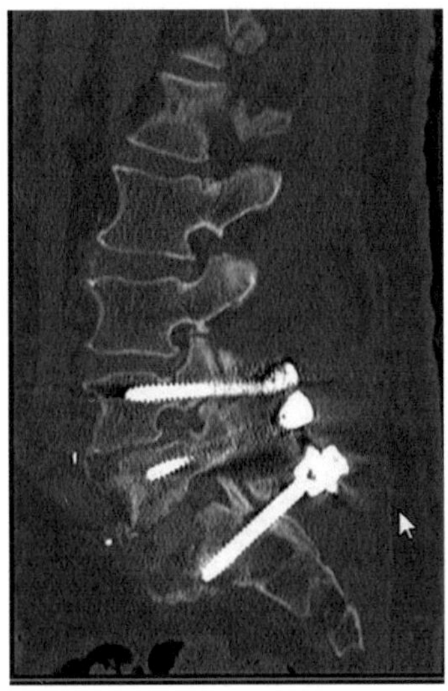

Figure 17.
Lumbar CT Sagittal 3month postoperative views demonstrating significant hardware lucency around the screws and the PEEK interbody cages.

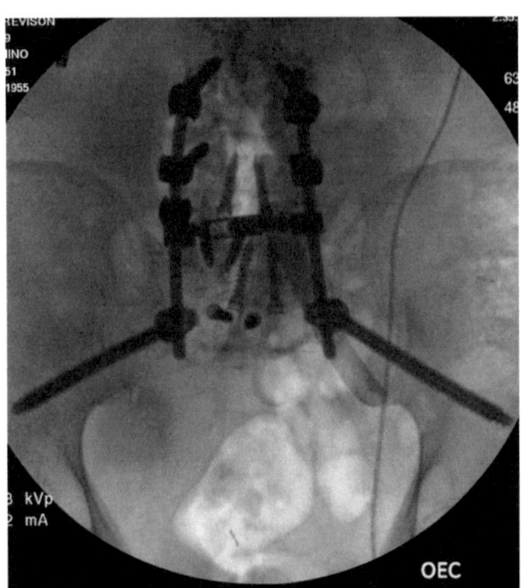

Figure 18.
Postoperative AP Demonstrating SAI screw fixation.

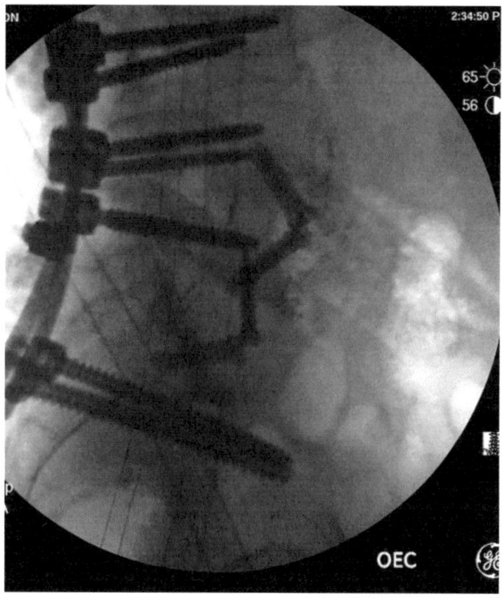

Figure 19.
Postoperative Lateral Imaging Demonstrating SAI screw fixation.

4. Conclusions

Sacral alar-iliac screws have been substantiated as a practical and effective means of achieving robust distal fixation when addressing situations ranging from revision surgery, fractures, tumor resection procedures, flat back deformity, paediatric and adult scoliosis. With properly indicated patients, meticulous preoperative planning, and sound surgical technique, sacroiliac screw fixation offers an excellent surgical option for many patients in need of distal fixation across the lumbosacral junction.

Conflict of interest

The author declares no current conflict of interest.

Author details

Pablo Pazmiño
SpineCal, Santa Monica, CA, USA

*Address all correspondence to: doctor@spinecal.com

References

[1] Hu X, Lieberman IH. Robotic-guided sacro-pelvic fixation using S2 alar-iliac screws: feasibility and accuracy. European Spine Journal. 2017;**26**(3):720-725

[2] Phan K, Li J, Giang G, Teng I, Phan S, Chang N, et al. A novel technique for placement of sacro-alar-iliac (S2AI) screws by K-wire insertion using intraoperative navigation. Journal of Clinical Neuroscience. 2017;**45**:324-327

[3] Mattei TA, Fassett DR. Combined S-1 and S-2 sacral alar-iliac screws as a salvage technique for pelvic fixation after pseudarthrosis and lumbosacropelvic instability: Technical note. Journal of Neurosurgery. Spine. 2013;**19**(3):321-330

[4] Park JH, Hyun SJ, Kim KJ, Jahng TA. Free hand insertion technique of S2 sacral alar-iliac screws for spino-pelvic fixation: Technical note, Acadaveric Study. Journal of Korean Neurosurgical Society. 2015;**58**(6):578-581

[5] Zhu F, Bao HD, Yuan S, Wang B, Qiao J, Zhu ZZ, et al. Posterior second sacral alar iliac screw insertion: anatomic study in a Chinese population. European Spine Journal. 2013;**22**(7):1683-1689

[6] Park SC, Hong TC, Yang JH, Chang DG, Suh SW, Nam Y, et al. Safe optimal tear drop view for spinopelvic fixation using a three-dimensional reconstruction model of the pelvis. Clinics in Orthopedic Surgery. 2023;**15**(3):436-443

Chapter 4

Adolescent Idiopathic Scoliosis

Shaker Barker

Abstract

Adolescent idiopathic scoliosis (AIS) is a common spinal disorder that primarily affects adolescents during their growth spurt. It is characterized by a lateral rotation curvature of the spine, typically in an "S" or "C" shape. The exact cause of this condition is still unknown, but it is believed to be influenced by a combination of genetic and environmental factors. Symptoms of adolescent idiopathic scoliosis may vary depending on the severity of the curvature, ranging from mild back pain to noticeable changes in posture. Early detection and intervention are essential to prevent further progression of the curve and to minimize potential complications. Treatment options include observation, bracing, and in severe cases, surgery. Regular monitoring and follow-up care are crucial in managing this condition and ensuring the overall well-being of affected individuals.

Keywords: spine, deformity, scoliosis, idiopathic, adolescence

1. Introduction

Scoliosis, a condition characterized by lateral curves in the vertebral column, affects spinal alignment in all three dimensions [1]. The term "scoliosis" originates from the ancient Greek word "skolios," meaning curved or crooked, and was first defined by Galen in the 2nd century AD [2]. There are various types of scoliosis categorized by factors like age of onset, cause, severity, and curvature type. Each type has distinct characteristics, including the rate of curve progression and the pattern of three-dimensional (3D) deformity [3]. The two main groups of scoliosis are idiopathic (unknown cause) and non-idiopathic. Idiopathic scoliosis is diagnosed when non-idiopathic causes are ruled out. Congenital scoliosis, on the other hand, is caused by vertebral malformations like hemivertebrae, unilateral web, or block vertebrae [4]. While not always noticeable at birth, it typically develops during adolescence. Both genetic and environmental factors can contribute to these malformations [5–7]. Scoliosis that is classified as neuromuscular is a result of weakened muscles that provide support for the spine. This type of scoliosis is commonly observed in individuals with conditions such as cerebral palsy, spinal muscular atrophy, spina bifida, muscular dystrophies, or spinal cord injuries [8]. On the other hand, mesenchymal scoliosis is caused by the weakening of passive stabilizers of the spine. This form of scoliosis is often present in individuals with conditions such as Marfan syndrome (**Figure 1**), [9] mucopolysaccharidosis, osteogenesis imperfecta, inflammatory diseases, or complications arising after surgery.

Infantile scoliosis, affecting children aged 0–3 years, has a prevalence rate of 1%. The recommendation for infants to be placed in the prone position during the 1980s resulted in a significant decrease in the number of cases [10, 11]. Unlike adolescent

IntechOpen

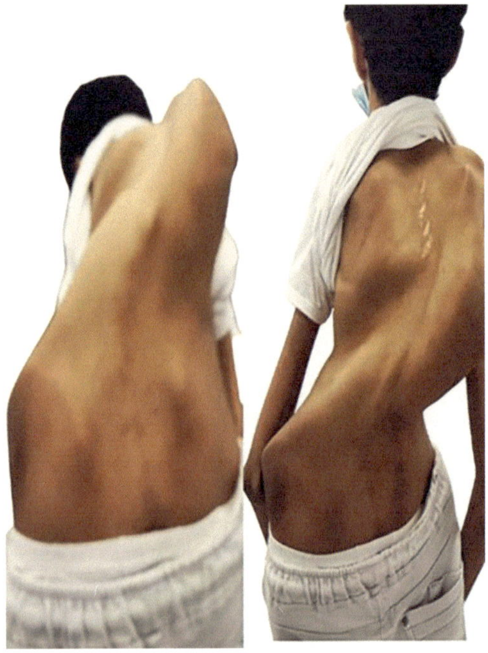

Figure 1.
Male 15 years old with triple curve scoliosis in Mar Fan Syndrome [9].

idiopathic scoliosis (AIS), more than half of the cases of infantile scoliosis regress over time [12]. When the rib-vertebrae angle (RVA) exhibits a difference of more than 20 degrees, it indicates a negative prognosis and a rapid advancement of the condition. Juvenile scoliosis, which typically manifests between the ages of 4 and 10, accounts for approximately 10–15% of all cases of idiopathic scoliosis in children. Failure to address this condition can result in severe complications related to the heart and lungs (**Figure 2**) [13]. It is worth noting that curvatures measuring 30 degrees or greater tend to worsen over time, leading to the necessity of surgical intervention in 95% of affected patients. Adolescent scoliosis, which typically arises in individuals aged 11–18 years, is a common form of scoliosis found in teenagers [14].

2. Etiology

Several studies suggest that genetic factors play a crucial role in the etiology of AIS. Familial aggregation and twin studies have provided evidence of heritability, indicating that there is a genetic predisposition to AIS [15, 16]. Genome-wide association studies (GWAS) have identified potential candidate genes associated with AIS, such as LBX1, GPR126, and PAX1 [17]. Polymorphisms in estrogen receptor genes have been linked to the risk of developing AIS, implying that hormonal imbalances could also be implicated in its etiology [18]. Despite these findings, the specific mechanisms by which these genetic factors contribute to the development of AIS are still not fully understood. Apart from genetic factors, non-genetic factors may also play a significant role in AIS etiology. Biomechanical factors, such as asymmetrical loading of the spine, abnormal spinal growth patterns, and imbalances in muscle tension, have been proposed as potential triggers of AIS [19]. These factors can lead to mechanical forces that disrupt the normal

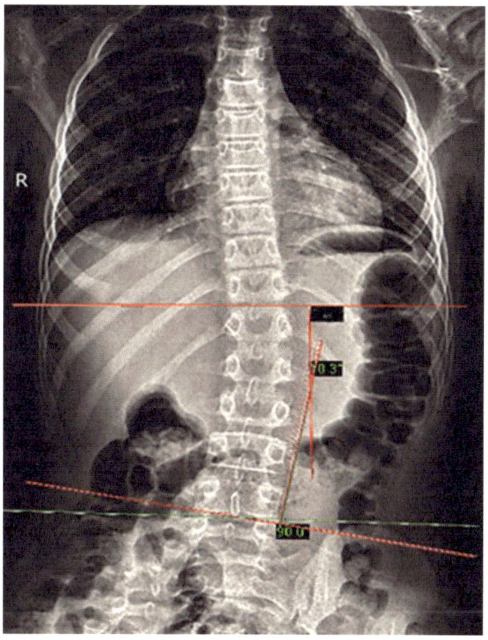

Figure 2.
Male 8 years old with lumbar juvenile scoliosis pelvic tile more than 1.5 degree and Cobb angel 10.3.

growth and development of the spine during adolescence, contributing to the onset of scoliosis. Additionally, neurologic abnormalities, including abnormal proprioception and impaired neuromuscular control, have been suggested to play a role in AIS etiology. Changes in the central nervous system's ability to control posture and muscular activation may result in abnormalities in spinal alignment and development [20–22]. Hormonal imbalances during adolescence have been implicated in the etiology of AIS. Estrogens, particularly 17β-estradiol, have been shown to influence bone growth and remodeling [23, 24]. Experimental studies have suggested that estrogen deficiency or altered estrogen signaling may disrupt the balance between bone formation and resorption, leading to structural abnormalities in the spine [23, 25]. However, the exact role of hormones in AIS etiology is still under investigation, and further research is required to establish a clear causative relationship.

3. Epidemiology

The frequency of AIS is approximately 1–3%. Prearrange female and the right-side curves. To be considered scoliosis, the degree of coronal plane's curvature must be more than 10°. For patients with curvatures that are greater than 40 degrees, the frequency is approximately 0.1% [26].

4. History

A comprehensive history and physical examination are necessary. Detailed developmental history to exclude other causes of scoliosis. Also, attention must be paid to questions pertaining to skeletal development, including the age of menarche. In a gross description, most adolescents with idiopathic scoliosis that present with no pain at the back will not have a dramatic reaction to the curvature. Many will participate in activities that are both physical and mental, including athletes, cheerleaders, and otherwise healthy children [27–29].

5. Physical examination

5.1 Assessment of shoulder tilt

Shoulder tilt can be assessed looking at the patient posteriorly as well as anteriorly. If one shoulder is higher than the other, it should be noted: larger space from arm to the side of the body when comparing both sides (**Figure 3**).

5.2 Assessment of pelvic tilt

The presence of asymmetry of waist crease, truncal shift, and pelvic tilt should also be assessed by direct visualization. One hip higher than the other; head not centered over pelvis uneven waist creases.

5.3 Assessment of angle of trunk rotation

A scoliometer is used to assess the angle of trunk rotation for the thoracic as well as the lumbar prominence while the patient is in a forward bending position in "Adam's forward test." (**Figure 4**).

5.4 Presence of any cutaneous abnormalities

The presence of cutaneous abnormalities, such as hairy spots or "café au lait" spots, can be a presence of non-idiopathic types of scoliosis and should be kept in mind [30].

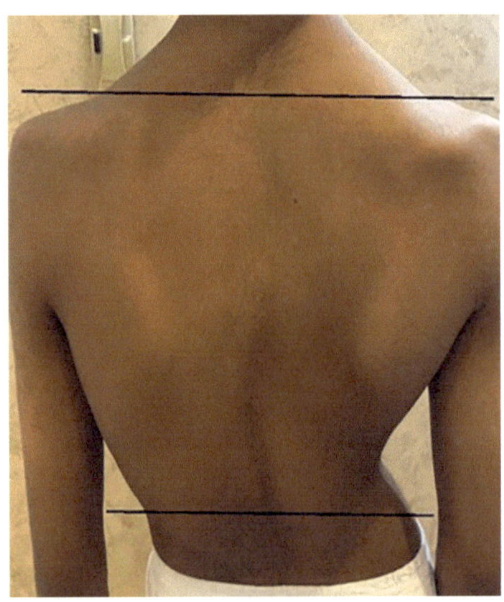

Figure 3.
Shoulder and pelvis tilts with waist creases.

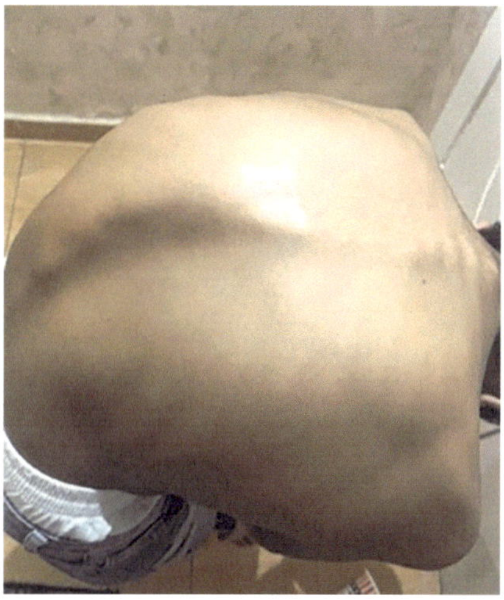

Figure 4.
Adam's forward test.

5.5 Indicators of maturity

Development of secondary sexual characteristics is a rough indication of skeletal maturity and should be kept in mind.

5.6 Gait assessment

It is important for indicating any leg length discrepancies or ataxia, which may be an indication of spinal cord disorders.

6. Radiological assessment

The formal evaluation that is proper includes X-ray imaging. Patients require a permanent coronal X-ray, a sagittal X-ray, a left and right bend X-ray. The Risser classification is typically derived from the iliac crest on a coronal X-ray view. Consensus is that a computed tomography (CT) scan and a magnetic resonance imaging (MRI) of the typical AIS patient are not necessary.

6.1 Essential radiographs

Radiologic analysis includes standing, long view of the spine, including the pelvis, to assess the Cobb angle (measured between the superior surface of the proximal and inferior surface of the distal end vertebrae tilted maximally into curvature) (**Figures 5** and **6**).

6.2 Flexibility views

Left and right bending view with the patient positioned supine (**Figures 7** and **8**) are obtained to determine the structural nature of the curve. Disc space neutralization defined as opening of the disc space across both sides on bending radiographs helps decide the distal extent of the fusion. These techniques are useful during surgical planning.

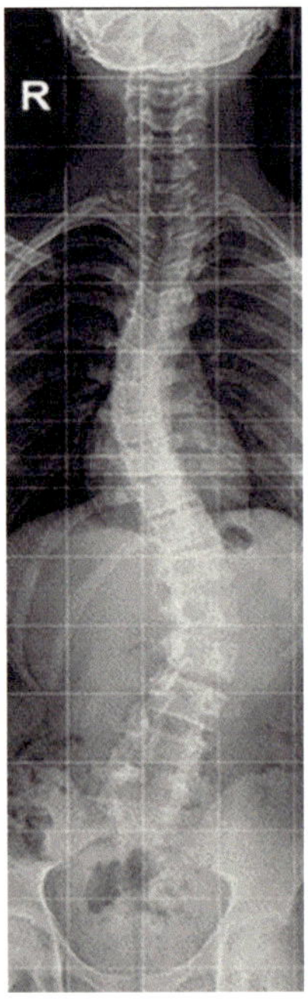

Figure 5.
Long view of the spine, including the pelvis.

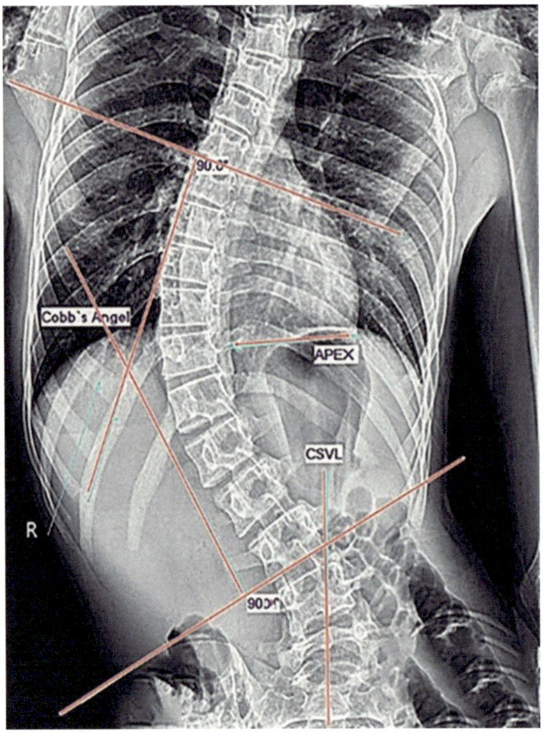

Figure 6.
Cobb angle (measured between the superior surface of the proximal and inferior surface of the distal end vertebrae tilted maximally into curvature).

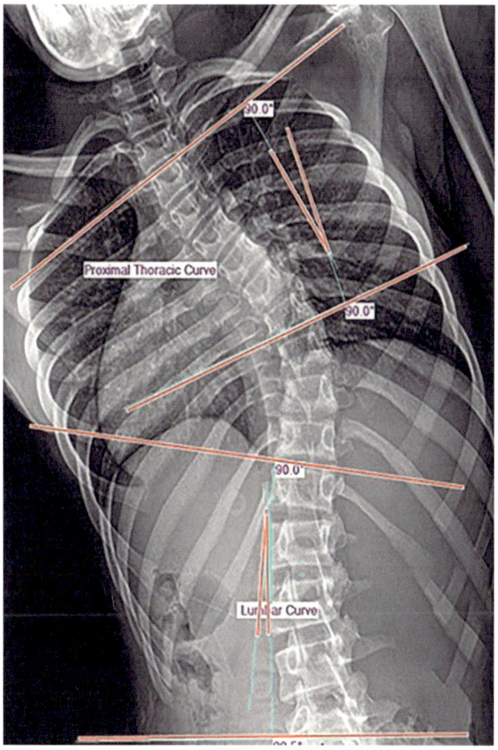

Figure 7.
Right bending view to measure the proximal thoracic and thoracolumbar/lumbar curves.

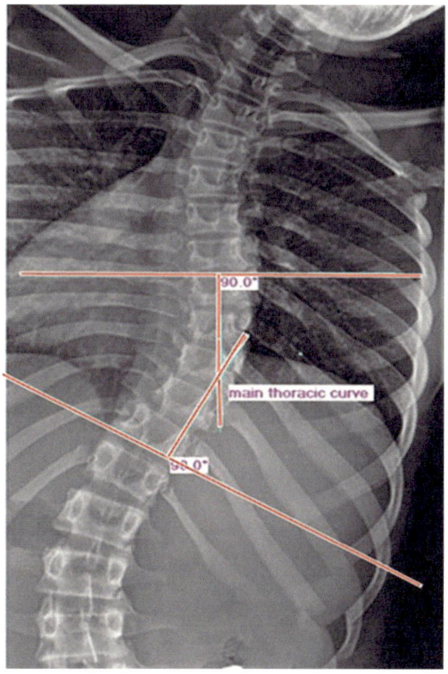

Figure 8.
Left bending view to measure main thoracic curve.

6.3 Lateral view

Cobb angles are measured in a more uniform fashion in the following way:

A. T2–T5

B. T5–T12

C. T10–L2

D. L1–S1

In the case of a severe kyphotic deformity, an additional measurement of maximal kyphosis can be used. The superior end-plate is used for the proximal end vertebra, while the inferior end-plate is used for the distal end vertebra to measure out the area of maximal kyphosis (**Figures 9** and **10**).

6.4 Skeletal maturity

The Risser Sign is a physical indicator used in orthopedics to measure the maturity of the pelvic bones in adolescents. To measure skeletal development, one can utilize the Risser sign, which only requires an X-ray of the pelvis. The X-ray reveals the ossification of the iliac apophysis as it advances from the crest toward the spine. The Risser sign is categorized into five different stages, with stage 1 indicating 25% ossification and occurring during early puberty. Once a person reaches Risser stage 5, their bones are fully ossified, and they are deemed to be skeletally mature.

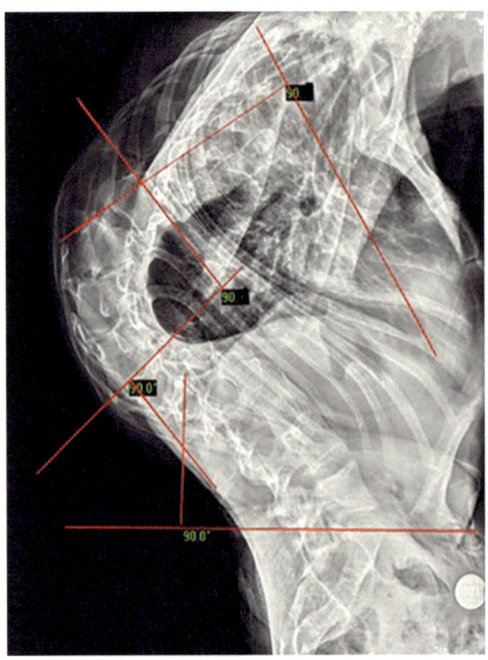

Figure 9.
Measure the maximal kyphosis case of scoliosis with severe kyphosis.

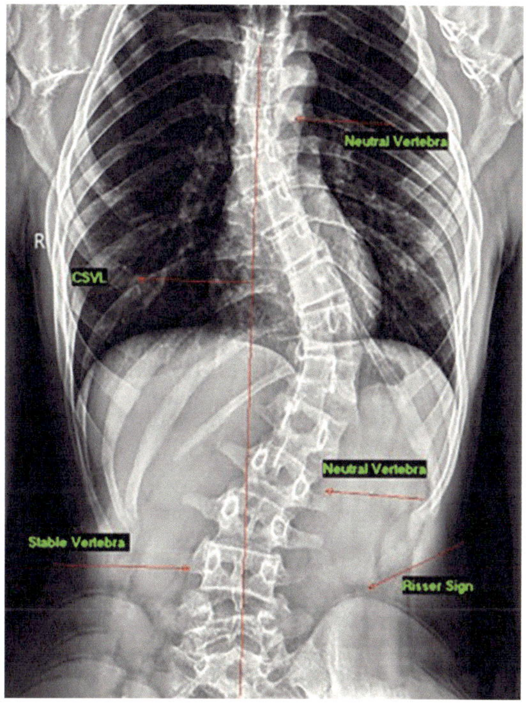

Figure 10.
Radiographic marker of CSVL; SV; NV; Risser Sign.

The Sanders Maturity Scale is a tool utilized to measure the maturity of an individual or group. A child's bone maturity can be evaluated by an X-ray of the fingers and wrist on the left hand, using what is known as the Sanders score. This score uses a scale of 1–8, with 1 signifying slow growth during early adolescence and 8 representing complete skeletal maturity. Recent studies have shown that the Sanders Maturity Scale is a more dependable metric for measuring skeletal maturity in patients with adolescent idiopathic scoliosis, particularly during the curve acceleration phase, as opposed to the Risser classification.

7. Diagnosis

The diagnosis of AIS remains a diagnosis of exclusion, and other probable causes of scoliosis, such as spinal infections and neoplasms, neuromuscular and syndromic diseases, and congenital anomalies of the spine or neural axis, should be excluded.

7.1 Staging

The Lenke System of AIS Classification is most effective at categorizing stages. The objective of this classification scheme is to create a common method of naming and describing curves. The overall goal at this advanced level is also to favor the protocol for operative treatment [31].

7.1.1 Lenke classification

The Lenke classification for AIS has gained popularity and consists of three steps:

1. curve type (1–6)

2. lumbar mixed spine modifier (A, B, C)

3. sagittal thoracic modifier (–, N, +)

7.1.1.1 Identification of primary curve (Type 1–6)

1. Measure regional curves

    - proximal thoracic (PT)

    - main thoracic (MT)

    - thoracolumbar/lumbar (TL/L)

7.1.1.2 Identify major curve (biggest curve)

- always either MT (Type 1–4) or.MT/L (Type 4*,5,6)

7.1.1.3 Determine if minor curve is structural or not

- definition of structural

- >25° in coronal plane on standing anteroposterior (AP) and do not bend out to <25° on bending views.

- OR > 20° in sagittal plane.

Structural (major) – has the largest Cobb angle and is always structural. In Type 4, it can be either MT or FL/L depending on which Cobb is larger, if is the largest curve, then by default assign major curve to MT (**Table 1**) [32].

Type	Curve	Proximal thoracic	Main thoracic	Thoracolumbar/ lumbar
1	Main thoracic	Not structural	Structural	Not structural
2	Double thoracic	Structural	Structural	Not structural
3	Double major	Not structural	Structural	Structural
4	Triple major	Structural	Structural	Structural
5	Thoracolumbar/lumbar	Not structural	Not structural	Structural
6	Thoracolumbar/lumbar-main thoracic	Structural	Structural	Structural

Table 1.
Description of Lenke classification.

7.1.1.4 Assignment of Lumbar modifiers (A, B, C)

- Identify apical lumbar vertebrae (ALV)
- is the inferior lumbar body that falls outside of the curve
- Draw central sacral vertical line (CSVL) and see where it sits in relationship to pedicles of ALV (**Table 2** and **Figure 11**) [32].

7.1.1.5 Assignment of sagittal thoracic modifier (–, N, +)

Measure sagittal Cobb from T5 to T12:
hypokyphotic (–) if <10°
normal if 10–40°
hyperkyphotic (+) if >40°

7.1.2 The three-dimensional classification system of scoliosis

The system for classifying scoliosis is based on its three-dimensional (3D) features. It was developed in 2001 by Dr. Lenke and colleagues at the University of Iowa (UI). The system is based on the following factors:

Modifiers			
Lumbar spine modifier	CSVL to lumbar apex	Thoracic sagittal profile	
A	CSVL between pedicles	– (below normal)	<10°
B	CSVL touches apical bodies	N (normal)	10°–40°
C	CSVL completely medial	+ (above normal)	>40°

A if CSVL passes between pedicles of apical lumbar vertebrae (ALV).
B modifier if CSVL touches the pedicle of apical lumbar vertebrae (ALV).
C modifier if CSVL does not touch apical lumbar vertebrae (ALV) apex of lumbar curve falls completely off the midline depicting a curve with complete apical translation off the CSVL.

Table 2.
Lumbar modifier of Lenke classification.

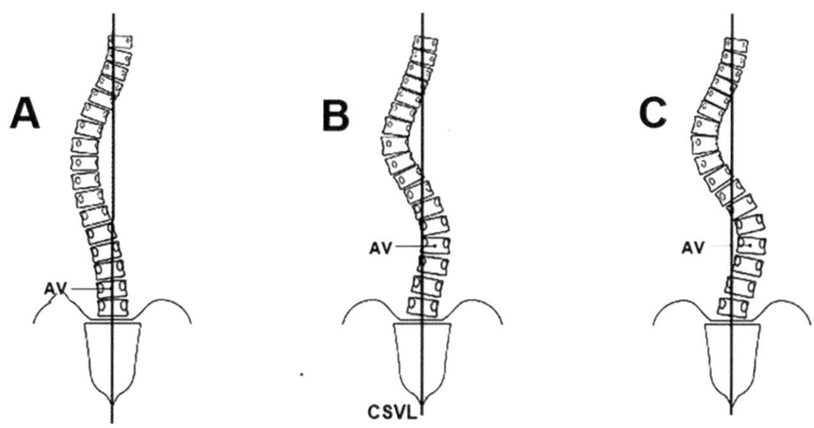

Figure 11.
Lumbar modifier Lenke Classification.

- The location of the curves in the coronal plane (front view)
- The location of the curves in the sagittal plane (side view)
- The flexibility of the curves
- The amount of rotation of the vertebrae

It is a more comprehensive system than previous systems, as it considers the 3D features of the curves. This allows surgeons to better plan treatment and predict the outcome of surgery.

Table 3 summarizes the different types of scoliosis in the Three-Dimensional Classification System:

The Three-Dimensional Classification System of scoliosis is a valuable tool for surgeons and other healthcare professionals who treat scoliosis. It provides a more comprehensive understanding of the deformity and helps to guide treatment decisions.

8. Treatment

The approach to treating AIS is contingent upon the severity of the curvature and factors such as the patient's age and growth status. In general, AIS curves advance in two distinct manners: first, during the rapid growth phase of the patient, and second, into adulthood if the trends are substantial. As scoliosis curves intensify during periods of growth, the potential for growth is evaluated by considering the patient's age, the onset of menstruation, and radiographic measurements. Typically, girls experience maturation around the age of 14, while boys reach maturity around the age of 16. Girls undergo rapid growth primarily during their initial menstrual cycle, which is then followed by a deceleration in growth. However, they will continue to grow

Type	Location of curves in coronal plane	Location of curves in sagittal plane	Flexibility of curves	Amount of rotation of vertebrae
Lenke 1	Single thoracic curve	Thoracic kyphosis	Flexible	Variable
Lenke 2	Double thoracic curves	Thoracic kyphosis	Flexible	Variable
Lenke 3	Thoracolumbar curve	Thoracic kyphosis or lordosis	Flexible or stiff	Variable
Lenke 4	Lumbar curve	Lumbar lordosis	Flexible or stiff	Variable
Lenke 5	Double major curves	Thoracic kyphosis or lordosis	Flexible or stiff	Variable
Lenke 6	Triple major curves	Thoracic kyphosis or lordosis	Flexible or stiff	Variable
Lenke 7	C curve	Variable	Variable	Variable
Lenke 8	Nonstructural curve	Variable	Variable	Variable
Lenke 9	Unclassified curve	Variable	Variable	Variable

Table 3.
Description of three-dimensional classification system of scoliosis.

for a period of 18 to 24 months after their first period. A widely employed method for evaluating the skeletal maturity of children, specifically the amount of growth remaining in the pelvis and spine, is the Risser system of grading (**Figure 8**). This system utilizes a scale ranging from 0 to 5 to determine the degree of skeletal maturation in a child. Patients classified as Risser 0 and 1 are still experiencing growth, whereas those categorized as Risser 4 and 5 have reached a point where growth has ceased. The three primary treatment options available include observation, bracing, and surgery (**Table 4**).

8.1 Observation

It is the most conservative approach to treatment. It's typically recommended for patients with curves of 10–25 degrees who are evaluated by means of serial X-rays. This is typically accomplished at 3, 6, or 12 monthly intervals [33].

8.2 Bracing

Those with a degree of curve greater than 25 but less than 40–45 are considered candidates for bracing. The Bracing in Adolescent Idiopathic Scoliosis Trial (BrAIST) was a National Institutes of Health (NIH)-funded experimental research trial that demonstrated the efficacy of bracing in the adolescent population. Despite the common usage of braces, these uncomfortable devices have a low rate of compliance, and their overall success is still debatable. Concerns have been expressed regarding every form of brace for dealing with scoliosis (**Figure 12**) [34, 35].

8.3 Surgery

When it comes to the treatment of scoliosis, surgery is considered the most drastic and intrusive option. Typically, it is advised for individuals with curves that exceed 45 degrees or those that are advancing rapidly [36–38]. Vertebral body tethering (VBT) is a non-fusion, compression-based, growth preserving alternative to posterior spinal fusion (PSF) based on the concept of "growth modulation" to prevent possible functional complications secondary to fusion while correcting scoliotic deformity. The surgical procedure. The goal of the procedure is to provide tension to the convexity of the thoracolumbar curve and thereby slow down the ipsilateral paraspinal musculature growth [39, 40]. When it comes to treating Type 1 curves, experts recommend

Treatment	Description	Advantages	Disadvantages
Observation	The patient is monitored regularly with X-rays to see if the curve progresses.	No side effects	Curve may progress.
Bracing	A brace is worn to help correct the curve.	Curve may be corrected or stabilized.	Brace can be uncomfortable and may not be effective for all patients.
Surgery	The spine is fused to straighten it.	Curve is corrected.	Surgery is invasive and has risks.

Table 4.
Treatment options of AIS.

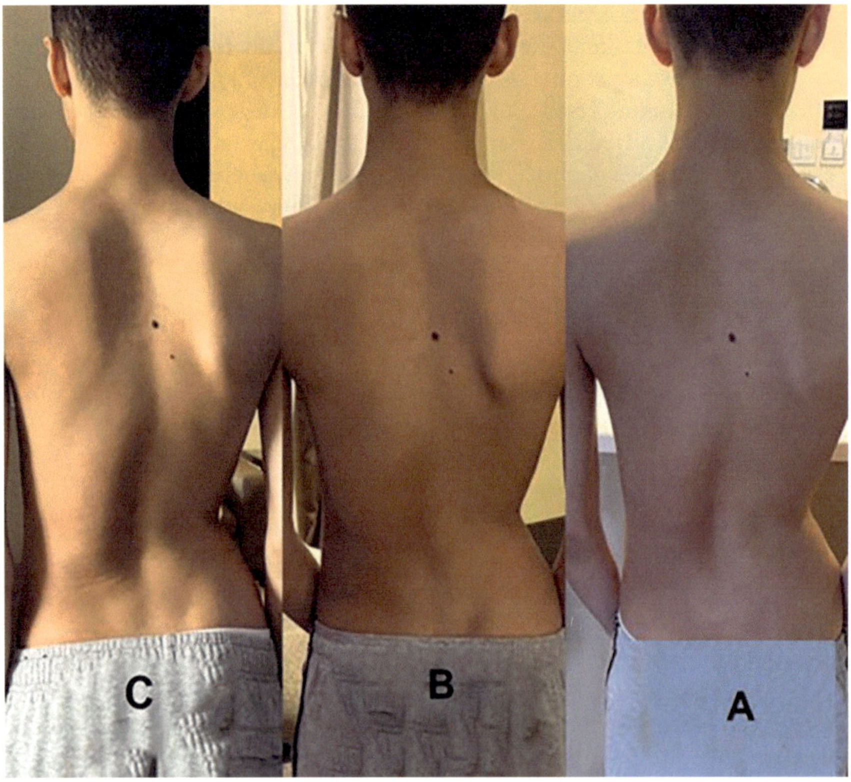

Figure 12.
Male 12 years old case of thoracolumbar AIS treated by physiotherapy and bracing for 9 months where A after 3: B after 6 and C after 9 months of treatment.

fusing the structural main thoracic curve. The UIV, or upper instrumented vertebra, typically falls between T3 and T5, while the LIV, or lowest instrumented vertebra, will vary depending on the location of both the stable and neutral vertebrae. The selection of the UIV considers shoulder balance as well as the presence of proximal thoracic kyphosis. It is important to avoid ending the construct at a region of kyphosis. For instance, if dealing with a right main thoracic curve and level shoulders, T3 would be the UIV of choice; however, T4 or T5 would be selected if the right shoulder was higher. The choice of LIV depends on the lumbar adjuster and CSVL. For lumbar adjusters A and B, the LIV can be selected as the heaviest lumbar vertebra that intersects the CSVL and is rotationally neutral. The LIV is usually located between the terminal and stabilizing vertebrae of the main thoracic curve. While not commonly observed in type 1 curves, T2 can be chosen as the upper instrumented vertebra (UIV) if the left shoulder is elevated higher than the right. Intraoperatively, the selection of the UIV may vary depending on the amount of main thoracic (MT) correction planned. The greater the correction planned, the likelier it is to fuse at a higher point in the proximal thoracic (PT) region to prevent the elevation of the opposite shoulder. The selection of the UIV can therefore be a dynamic process that is adjusted according to the amount of correction needed.

The determination of the most suitable treatment for a specific patient is a collaborative effort involving a healthcare team consisting of a physician, a physical therapist, and an expert in scoliosis braces. Factors, such as the patient's age, growth status, severity of the curve, and other relevant considerations, are considered to provide a personalized recommendation [41].

9. Prevention

Early detection and intervention play a crucial role in managing AIS effectively. Regular screenings in schools and healthcare settings can help identify the condition early, allowing for timely intervention and preventing the progression of the curve. If left untreated, AIS can lead to various complications, such as chronic pain, respiratory problems, and psychological distress, due to body image concerns. Early initiation of treatment can significantly improve the long-term outcomes and quality of life for individuals with AIS.

Conflict of interest

The authors declare no conflict of interest.

Declaration of figures' authenticity

All figures submitted have been created by the authors who confirm that the images are original with no duplication and have not been previously published in whole or in part.

List of abbreviations

AIS	adolescent idiopathic scoliosis
RVA	rib-vertebra angle
GWAS	genome-wide association studies
PA View	posterior–anterior view
NV	neutral vertebra
SV	stable vertebra
CSVL	central sacrum vertical line
PTC	proximal thoracic curve
MTC	main thoracic curve
TLC	thoracolumbar curve
LC	lumbar curve
SRS	Scoliosis Research Society
ALV	apical lumbar vertebra
UI	University of Iowa
BrAIST	The Bracing in Adolescent Idiopathic Scoliosis Trial

Author details

Shaker Barker
Saudi Spine Society, Balgsoon Medical Center, Jeddah, Saudi Arabia

*Address all correspondence to: shaker.barker@outlook.sa

References

[1] Morrissy RT, Weinstein SL. Lovell and Winter's Pediatric Orthopaedics. Philadelphia: Lippincott Williams & Wilkins; 2006. pp. 693-762

[2] Withington ET. Hippocrates on Joints 47 (Loeb Vol. 3). London: William Heinemann; 1928. pp. 297-299

[3] Campbell RM Jr, Hell-Vocke AK. Growth of the thoracic spine in congenital scoliosis after expansion thoracoplasty. The Journal of Bone and Joint Surgery. American Volume. 2003;**85-A**(3):409-420

[4] Mc M. Congenital scoliosis. In: Weinstein SL, editor. The Pediatric Spine: Principles and Practices. New York: Raven Press; 1994. pp. 227-244

[5] Bulman MP, Kusumi K, Frayling TM, et al. Mutations in the human delta homologue, DLL3, cause axial skeletal defects in spondylocostal dysostosis. Nature Genetics. 2000;**24**:438-441

[6] Li L, Krantz ID, Deng Y, et al. Alagille syndrome is caused by mutations in human jagged 1, which encodes a ligand for Notch 1. Nature Genetics. 1997;**16**:243-251

[7] Oda T, Elkahloun AG, Pike BL, et al. Mutations in the human jagged1 gene are responsible for Alagille syndrome. Nature Genetics. 1997;**16**:235-242

[8] Reames DL, Smith JS, Fu KM, Polly DW Jr, Ames CP, Berven SH, et al. Complications in the surgical treatment of 19,360 cases of pediatric scoliosis: A review of the Scoliosis Research Society Morbidity and mortality database. Spine (Phila Pa 1976). 2011;**36**(18):1484-1491

[9] Barker SA. Trible curve scoliosis with acetabula protrusion in Marfan syndrome. MAR Orthopedics. 2023;**4**(6):1

[10] Mau H. The changing concept of infantile scoliosis. International Orthopaedics. 1981;**5**:131-137

[11] McMaster M. Infantile idiopathic scoliosis: Can it be prevented? Journal of Bone and Joint Surgery. British Volume (London). 1983;**65**:612-617

[12] Mehta MH. The rib-vertebra angle in the early diagnosis between resolving and progressive infantile scoliosis. Journal of Bone and Joint Surgery. British Volume (London). 1972;**54**(2):230-243

[13] Coillard C, Circo AB, Rivard CH. SpineCor treatment for juvenile idiopathic scoliosis: SOSORT award 2010 winner. Scoliosis. 2010;**5**:25

[14] Fruergaard S, Ohrt-Nissen S, Dahl B, Kaltoft N, Gehrchen M. Neural axis abnormalities in patients with adolescent idiopathic scoliosis: Is routine magnetic resonance imaging indicated irrespective of curve severity? Neurospine. 2019;**16**(2):339-346

[15] Staub HA. Eine skoliotikerfamilie. Ein Beitrag zur Frage der kongenitalen Skoliose und der Hereditat der Skoliosen. Z. Orthop. Chir. 1922;**43**:1

[16] Horton D. Common skeletal deformities. In: Rimoin DL, Conner MJ, Pyeritz RE, Korf BR, editors. Emery & Rimoins Principles and Practices of Medical Genetics. Amsterdam: Churchill Livingstone Elsevier; 2002. pp. 4236-4244

[17] Zhu Z et al. Genome-wide association study identifies new susceptibility loci

for adolescent idiopathic scoliosis in Chinese girls. Nature Communications. 2015;**6**:8355. DOI: 10.1038/ncomms9355

[18] Alwan M et al. Archives of Razi Institute. 2022;**77**(3):943-958

[19] Stokes IA, Burwell RG, Dangerfield PH, IBSE. Biomechanical spinal growth modulation and progressive adolescent scoliosis – A test of the 'vicious cycle' pathogenetic hypothesis: Summary of an electronic focus group debate of the IBSE. Scoliosis. Oct 2006;**18**(1):16. DOI: 10.1186/1748-7161-1-16

[20] Le Febvre J, Triboulet-Chassevant A, Missirliu MF. Lerique and Le Coeur Electromyographic data in idiopathic scoliosis. Archives of Physical Medicine and Rehabilitation. 1961;**42**:710-711

[21] Riddle HF, Roaf R. Muscle imbalance in the causation of scoliosis. Lancet. 1955;**268**(6877):1245-1247. DOI: 10.1016/S0140-6736(55)91020-5

[22] Henssge J. Are signs of denervation of muscles of the spine primary or secondary findings in cases of scoliosis? Journal of Bone and Joint Surgery. 1968;**50B**:882-886

[23] Esposito T, Uccello R, Caliendo R, Di Martino GF, Gironi Carnevale UA, Cuomo S, et al. Estrogen receptor polymorphism, estrogen content and idiopathic scoliosis in human: A possible genetic linkage. The Journal of Steroid Biochemistry and Molecular Biology. 2009;**116**(1-2):56-60. DOI: 10.1016/j.jsbmb.2009.04.010

[24] Pöllänen E, Sipilä S, Alen M, Ronkainen PH, Ankarberg-Lindgren C, Puolakka J, et al. Differential influence of peripheral and systemic sex steroids on skeletal muscle quality in pre- and postmenopausal women. Aging Cell. 2011;**10**(4):650-660. DOI: 10.1111/j.1474-9726.2011.00701.x

[25] Skogland LB, Miller JA. Growth related hormones in idiopathic scoliosis. An endocrine basis for accelerated growth. Acta Orthopaedica Scandinavica. 1980;**51**(5):779-780. DOI: 10.3109/17453678008990874

[26] Rogala EJ, Drummond DS, Gurr J. Scoliosis: Incidence and natural history. A prospective epidemiological study. The Journal of Bone and Joint Surgery. American Volume. 1978;**60**:173-176

[27] Yagci G, Yakut Y. Core stabilization exercises versus scoliosis-specific exercises in moderate idiopathic scoliosis treatment. Prosthetics and Orthotics International. 2019;**43**(3):301-308

[28] Levi D, Springer S, Parmet Y, Ovadia D, Ben-Sira D. Acute muscle stretching and the ability to maintain posture in females with adolescent idiopathic scoliosis. Journal of Back and Musculoskeletal Rehabilitation. 2019;**32**(4):655-662

[29] van den Bogaart M, van Royen BJ, Haanstra TM, de Kleuver M, Faraj SSA. Predictive factors for brace treatment outcome in adolescent idiopathic scoliosis: A best-evidence synthesis. European Spine Journal. 2019;**28**(3):511-525

[30] Riccardi V. Neurofibromatosis. In: Neurologic Clinics, Neurocutaneous Disorders. 3rd ed. Vol. 5. Philadelphia: W.B. Saunders; 1987. pp. 337-349

[31] Lenke LG, Betz RR, Bridwell KH, Clements DH, Harms J, Lowe TG, et al. Intraobserver and interobserver reliability of the classification of thoracic adolescent idiopathic scoliosis. The Journal of Bone and Joint Surgery. American Volume. 1998;**80**:1097-1106

[32] Slattery C, Verma K. Classifications in brief: The Lenke classification for adolescent idiopathic scoliosis. Clinical Orthopaedics and Related Research. 2018;**476**(11):2271-22768. DOI: 10.1097/CORR.0000000000000405

[33] Stone B, Beekman C, Hall V, Guess V, Brooks HL. The effect of an exercise program on change in curve in adolescents with minimal idiopathic scoliosis. Physical Therapy. 1979;**59**:759-763

[34] Negrini S, Minozzi S, Bettany-Saltikov J, Zaina F, Chokalingam N, Grivas TB, et al. Braces for idiopathic scoliosis in adolescents. Spine (Phila Pa 1976). 2010;**35**:1285-1293

[35] Watts HG, Hall JE, Stanish W. The Boston brace system for the treatment of low thoracic and lumbar scoliosis by use of girdle without superstructure. Clinical Orthopaedics and Related Research. 1977;**126**:87-92

[36] Lonstein JE, Carlson JM. The prediction of curve progression in untreated idiopathic scoliosis during growth. The Journal of Bone and Joint Surgery. American Volume. 1984;**66**:1060-1071

[37] Weinstein SL, Ponseti IV. Curve progression in idiopathic scoliosis: Long term followup. The Journal of Bone and Joint Surgery. American Volume. 1983;**65**:447-455

[38] Edgar MA, Mehta MH. Long-term follow-up of fused and unfused idiopathic scoliosis. Journal of Bone and Joint Surgery. British Volume (London). 1988;**70**:712-716

[39] Hibbs RA. A report of 59 cases of scoliosis treated by the fusion operation. Journal of Bone and Joint Surgery. 1924;**6**:3-37

[40] Albee FH. Transplantation of a portion of tibia into the spine for Pott's disease. A preliminary report. Journal of the American Medical Association. 1911;**57**:885-886

[41] Sud A, Tsirikos AI. Current concepts and controversies on adolescent idiopathic scoliosis: Part I. Indian Journal of Orthopedics. 2013;**47**(2):117-128. DOI: 10.4103/0019-5413.108875

Chapter 5

Evaluation and Treatment of Cervical Spine Deformity

Weiye Zhang, Wei Tan, Samer G. Zammar, Kathryn Park, Justin Scheer, Young Lee, Alysha Jamison and Lee A. Tan

Abstract

The cervical spine plays a pivotal role in activities of daily living by allowing a wide range of motion while supporting the cranium. Cervical spine deformity (CSD) can cause significant negative impact on the patient's functional status and quality of life. Surgical correction of cervical spine deformity can be challenging due to the complexity of the regional neurovascular anatomy, which necessitates a comprehensive understanding of the cervical spine anatomy and biomechanics. Goals of cervical deformity surgery include decompression of neural elements, and restoration of cervical alignment, and achieving solid arthrodesis. Cervical spine deformity correction can involve various anterior and posterior surgical techniques. Careful surgical planning and meticulous surgical techniques are essential to minimize complications and optimize clinical outcomes in cervical deformity correction. In this chapter, we provide an in depth review of pre-operative evaluation, surgical planning, and treatment strategies for cervical spine deformity.

Keywords: cervical spine deformity, cervical alignment, anterior cervical osteotomy, Smith-Petersen osteotomy, pedicle subtraction osteotomy, complication avoidance

1. Introduction

The cervical spine is a highly mobile segment of the spinal column with the important role of supporting the weight of the head, maintain a horizontal gaze and allowing for a wide range of physical activities. Cervical deformity can cause significant disability and dysfunction, and has been correlated with poor health-related quality of life (HRQOL) [1–6], as well as ranked in the bottom 25th percentile of the EuroQol-5 Dimension (EQ-5D) HRQOL metric, along with heart failure, stroke, renal failure, emphysema, blindness, breast and prostate cancer when compared to other serious chronic diseases [7].

With an aging population and growing focus on cervical spine disorders and their impact on patient outcomes, utilization of cervical spine decompression and fusion procedures in the United States has been steadily rising each year [8]. Over the past decade, substantial progress has been made in the diagnosis and treatment of cervical deformities in adults. Established parameters now define both normal and pathological cervical alignment, and classification systems for cervical deformities, along with a cervical osteotomy classification, has been introduced [9–17]. Despite an increase in the cervical deformity knowledge base, this work is ever expanding and continues to evolve. The consolidation of the most relevant and clinically applicable information for adult cervical deformity is needed to aid the practicing surgeon as well as those in training to better understand and treat these complex patients and ultimately improve the clinical outcome.

In this chapter, we provide a comprehensive review of cervical biomechanics, radiographic alignment parameters, deformity classification, clinical evaluation, and pre-surgical planning, surgical techniques, and complication avoidance.

2. Cervical spine biomechanics

The primary function of the cervical spine is to support the head's position above the body and facilitate a level horizontal gaze. To accomplish this, the cervical spine has six distinct degrees of freedom in its movement. These encompass flexion/extension, axial rotation, and lateral bending, in addition to minor anterior/posterior translational movements along the Cartesian coordinates [18]. The head's center of mass (COM) is situated slightly above and forward of the external auditory canal, approximately 1 cm above the occipital condyle [19]. Any deviations from the typical cervical alignment that lead to a displacement of the head's center of mass result in an elevated cantilever load on the cervical spine. Consequently, this provokes an increased expenditure of energy by the paraspinal muscles [15]. Within the neutral zone of movement, the cervical spine can move with minimal energy demand from the paraspinal muscles. However, any motion beyond this neutral zone necessitates a greater force and energy input to overcome the elastic forces of the surrounding tissues. This region outside the neutral zone is aptly referred to as the elastic zone [18]. The physiologically accepted global ROM of the cervical spine typically encompasses approximately 90° of flexion, 70° of extension, 20° to 45° of lateral bending, and a maximum of 90° of rotation on each side [18, 20].

The atlanto-occipital and atlanto-axial joints unique joints of the cervical spine and because of their anatomy, they allow for significant specific motion at these segments. The atlanto-occipital joint is a synovial joint composed of the interface between the convex shaped occipital condyles and the concave shaped superior articular process of C1 [18]. This type of joint anatomy results in a large amount of flexion/extension, however, there is very little lateral bending movement or axial rotation [21]. In contrast, the atlanto-axial joint consists of four synovial joint interfaces. These include: the anterior arch of C1 and the odontoid process, the odontoid process and the transverse ligament, and the bilateral C1-2 articular surfaces. This type of joint results in a significant amount of axial rotation, but with more limited flexion/extension and lateral bending [18]. A study by Panjabi et al. [22] demonstrated that the flexion, extension, lateral bending, and axial rotation ROMS were the following: 3.5°, 21.0°, 5.5°, and 7.2°, respectively, at the atlanto-occipital joint, and 11.5°, 10.9°, 6.7°, and 38.9°, respectively, at the atlantoaxial joint. Therefore, the largest ROM between two cervical vertebral segments is the axial rotation at the atlantoaxial joint, with a neutral zone of 29.6° resulting in 75% of this motion.

The initial transfer of the axial load stemming from the weight of the head commences with its transmission from the occipital condyles to the lateral masses of C1. It subsequently progresses to the C1-2 facet joints, then to the lateral masses of C2, and ultimately disperses throughout the remainder of the spinal column by way of the intervertebral disc at C2-3 and the facet joints. This load is further distributed via the C2 articular pillars to engage the anterior column, the C2-3 disc, the posterior column, and the C2-3 facet [23]. The posterior columns of the cervical spine mostly handle the load distribution with 36% in the anterior column and 64% in the two posterior columns [23]. This is in contrast with the lumbar spine where the anterior loads 67–82% have been reported as higher than the posterior loads 18–33% [24, 25]. To counterbalance the thoracic spine's inherent kyphotic curvature, the cervical spine typically has a lordotic shape in the neutral position [26]. The lower part of the cervical spine, characterized by its lordotic curvature, meets the inflexible kyphotic thoracic inlet at the cervicothoracic junction (CTJ). Deviations from the normal cervical lordosis, such as the emergence of cervical kyphosis, are linked to pain and diminished functionality [6, 26–29]. In the presence of cervical kyphotic deformity, the center of mass (COM) of the head shifts forward, resulting in the formation of a lever arm, thereby generating a greater bending force [18]. The resulting increased bending force necessitates heightened contraction of the paraspinal muscles to uphold the head's upright position and sustain a level horizontal gaze. As previously noted, this heightened muscle effort can lead to muscle fatigue and discomfort [18]. Furthermore, a cervical kyphotic deformity will shift the forward movement of the head's axial load, which has the potential to expedite cervical disc degeneration. Additionally, a reduction in disc height due to degenerative changes can, in turn, exacerbate cervical kyphosis [18]. Moreover, pronounced cervical kyphosis can potentially cause elongation of the spinal cord, leading to heightened intramedullary pressure and compromised microcirculation. This, over time, can progress to spinal cord ischemia and subsequent myelopathy, as elaborated upon later. Nevertheless, it's crucial to note that not all instances of cervical kyphosis are classified as deformities, as many of them are symptomatic. Estimates suggest that cervical kyphosis can be observed in 2–35% of asymptomatic individuals [30–32].

3. Cervical alignment radiogrpahic measurements

3.1 Cervical radiographic alignment parameters

Cervical lordosis (CL) is an important cervical alignment parameter. There are three methods to measure CL and they include Cobb angles, Jackson's physiologic stress lines, and the Harrison posterior tangent method (**Figure 1**) [33].

The Cobb angle measurement technique entails drawing a line that is either parallel to the lower endplate of C2 or extending from the anterior tubercle of C1 to the posterior edge of the spinous process. Simultaneously, another line is drawn parallel to the lower endplate of C7. To determine the angle, perpendicular lines are then drawn from each of the aforementioned lines, and the cervical lordosis angle is measured as the angle formed where these perpendicular lines intersect [33]. The Jackson's physiologic stress lines method involves drawing a parallel line perpendicular to the posterior surface of each of the C7 and C2 vertebral bodies and calculating the angle between them [34]. Lastly, the Harrison posterior tangent method requires drawing lines that are parallel to the posterior surfaces of all cervical vertebral bodies from C2 to C7. The individual segmental angles are then summed to derive an overall cervical lordosis angle [35]. In the sagittal plane, the translation of the cervical spine is primarily assessed using cSVA. cSVA can be regionally defined as the distance

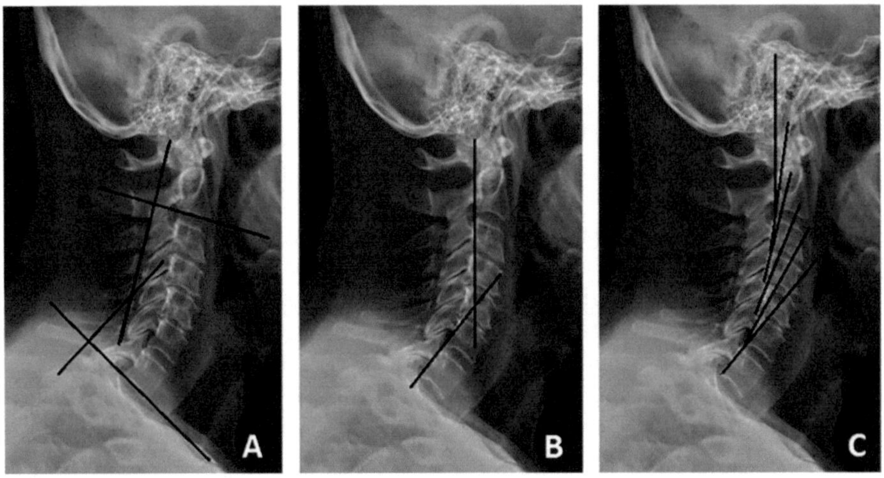

Figure 1.
Shows the three different ways to measure the cervical lordosis (CL). A) the cobb method involves drawing two parallel lines paths: The first runs parallel to the base of the second cervical vertebra (C-2), and the second parallel to the lower edge of the seventh cervical vertebra (C-7). Next, lines perpendicular to the first two are drawn, and the point where these perpendicular lines intersect determines the cervical curvature's angle. B) Jackson's physiological stress line technique involves sketching a pair of lines parallel to the posterior surfaces of the C-7 and C-2 vertebrae. Subsequently, the angle formed by these two lines is precisely measured. C) Harrison's posterior tangent approach: This method involves tracing lines parallel to the posterior surfaces of each cervical vertebra, from C-2 to C-7. The individual segmental angles are then summed up to calculate the total curvature angle of the neck.

between a plumb line dropped from the centroid of C2 and the superior posterior aspect of the C7 vertebral body (refer to **Figure 2**).

An alternative approach to evaluating global sagittal alignment is the use of the gravity line, measured from the center of gravity (COG) of the head, alongside the C7 plumb line (COG SVA) [36–42] This method can also be applied regionally for cervical SVA by drawing a plumb line from the center of gravity of the head instead of C2 (COG-C7 SVA). On lateral radiographs, approximating the center of gravity of the head can be achieved by initiating the plumb line at the anterior part of the external auditory canal [19]. However, it's worth noting that the C2 plumb line holds particular clinical significance, as it has a direct correlation with Health-Related Quality of Life (HRQOL), with larger C2 SVA values associated with poorer HRQOL [6].

For the measurement of horizontal gaze, the chin-brow-vertical-angle (CBVA) is employed. This measurement proves especially valuable in the management of severe, rigid cervical kyphotic deformities, as the loss of horizontal gaze significantly impacts daily activities and overall quality of life [43]. The CBVA is defined as the angle formed between a line drawn from the patient's chin to brow and a vertical line (refer to **Figure 3**).

The angle is assessed using clinical photographs of the patient standing with their hips and knees extended, maintaining a neutral or fixed neck position [43]. Notably, deformity correction that takes into account the chin-brow-vertical-angle (CBVA) has demonstrated a significant connection with favorable postoperative results, including enhanced gaze, walking ability, and daily activities [43–48]. A contemporary and highly significant parameter for evaluating cervical alignment is the T1 slope. This angle is defined as the measurement formed between a line parallel to the superior endplate of T1 and a horizontal reference line (refer to **Figure 4**).

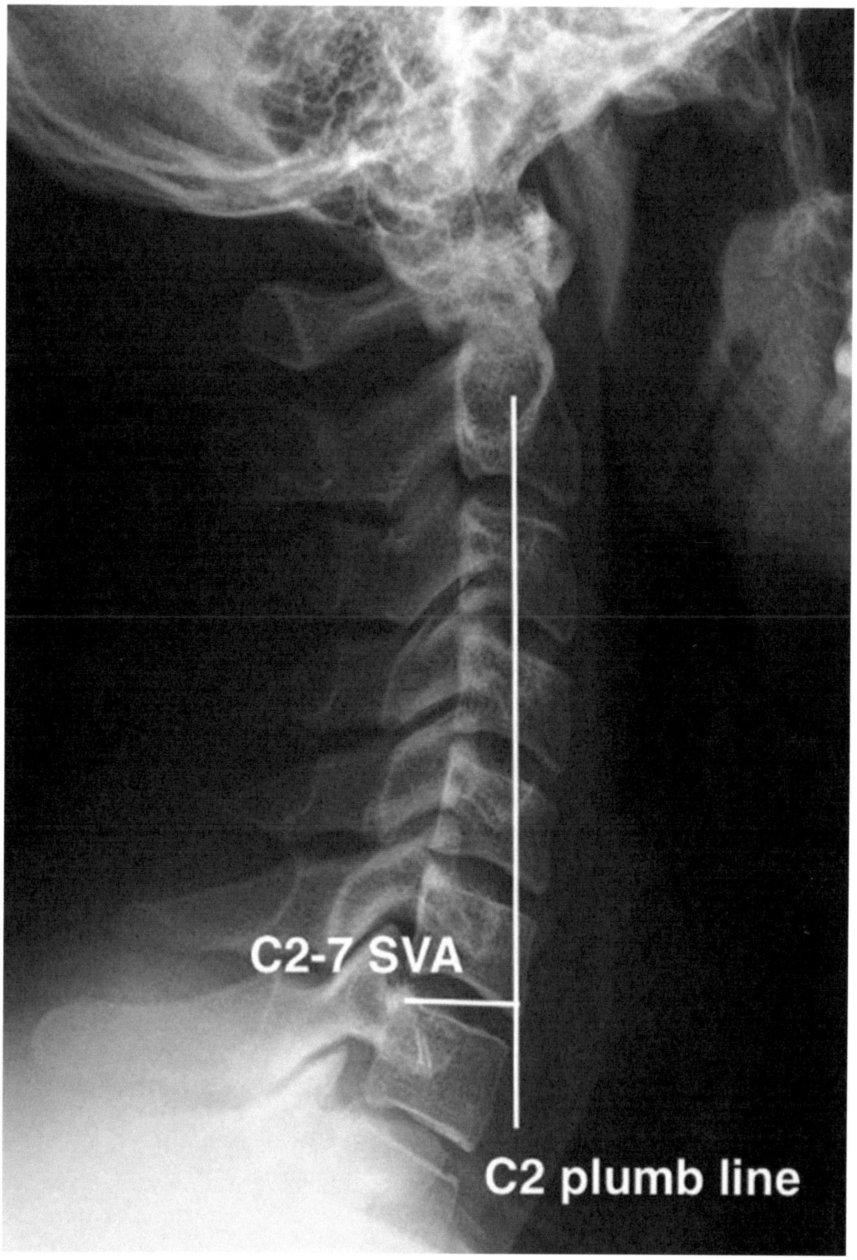

Figure 2.
C2-7 SVA defined as the distance from the superior posterior edge of C7 vertebral body to the C2 plumb line.

Once the T1S angle is determined, it becomes possible to calculate the discrepancy between CL and T1S, denoted as CL-T1S. Schwab and colleagues have highlighted that an individual's optimal lumbar lordosis (LL) should ideally fall within 10° of the pelvic incidence (PI), signified as LL = PI ± 10° [49, 50] A PI-LL mismatch exceeding 10° has been associated with notably inferior Health-Related Quality of Life (HRQOL), encompassing increased pain and disability, particularly among adults with thoracolumbar deformities [50–52]. In the cervical spine, a higher T1 slope necessitates

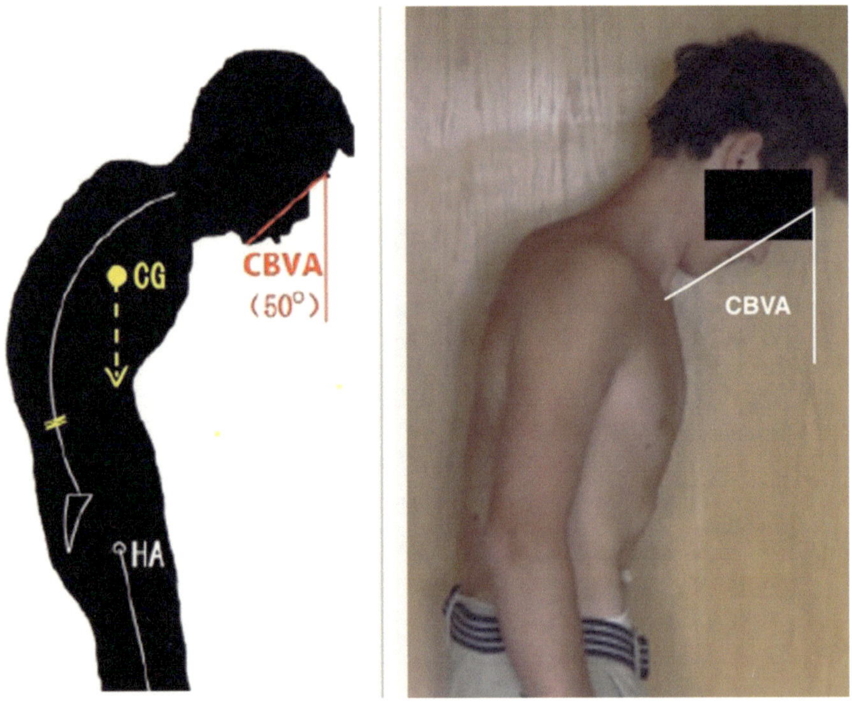

Figure 3.
The CBVA is defined as the angle formed between a line drawn from the patient's chin to brow and a vertical line.

a greater degree of cervical lordosis to achieve equilibrium in positioning the head over the thoracic inlet and trunk [15, 53]. This is akin to the concept of the mismatch between pelvic incidence and lumbar lordosis. In the cervical spine, this mismatch between T1 slope and cervical lordosis is termed TS-CL and has been proposed as a comparable parameter to the PI-LL mismatch [54, 55].

3.2 Normal cervical alignment

A broad spectrum of normal alignment has been documented, attributable to the cervical spine's remarkable mobility, as outlined in **Tables 1** and **2** [28, 29, 31, 56]. Among asymptomatic individuals, approximately 75–80% of cervical standing lordosis is concentrated within the C1-C2 segment [28, 57] while lower cervical levels exhibit comparatively less lordosis. This distribution mirrors the lumbar spine, where the preponderance of lumbar lordosis is concentrated at the caudal end, with L5-S1 featuring the most significant segmental lordotic angle [58]. The predominance of cervical lordosis in the C1-C2 region can be elucidated by the findings of Beier et al. [19] which indicate that the head's center of gravity aligns closely with the centers of the C1 and C2 vertebral bodies. On average, the total cervical lordosis measures approximately −40 degrees, with the occiput-C1 segment typically displaying a kyphotic curve [28]. Merley 6 degrees (15%) of lordosis occurs at the lowest three cervical levels (C4-C7) [28]. In terms of total cervical lordosis, there is no discernible difference between asymptomatic men and women, and there exists a positive correlation between cervical lordosis and advancing age [28, 31]. The average distance for cSVA falls within the range of 15–17 ± 11.2 mm, while the characterization of normal

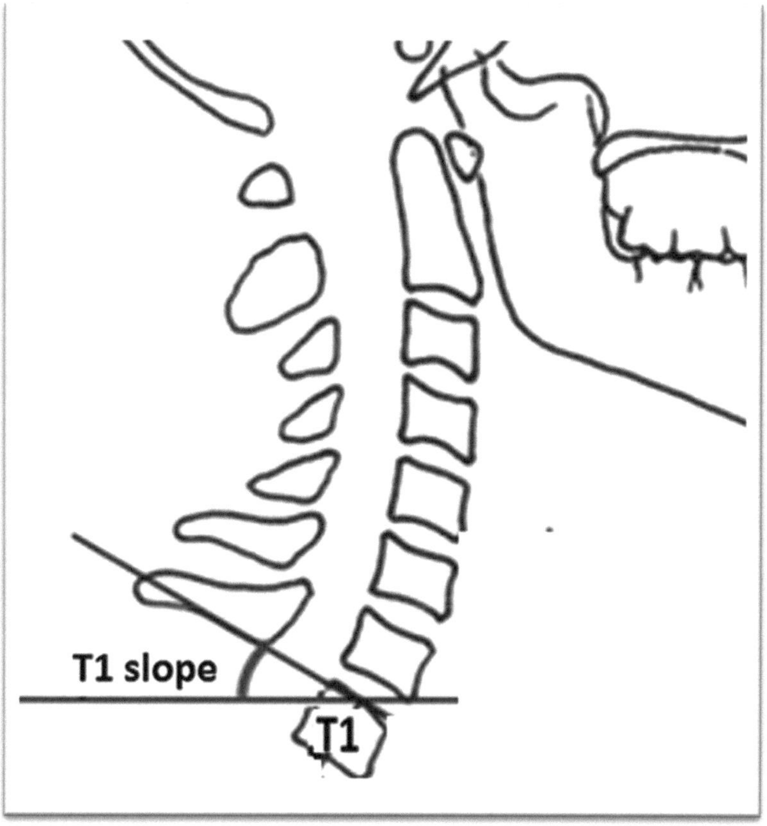

Figure 4.
T1 slope is defined as the measurement formed between a line parallel to the superior endplate of T1 and a horizontal reference line.

CBVA remains undefined. However, postoperative values ranging from +10 to −10 degrees have been well tolerated by patients [43–48].

Cervical lordosis seems to be intricately linked to the anatomy of the cervicothoracic junction (CTJ), typically encompassing C7 and T1 vertebrae, the C1-C7 disc, and the surrounding ligaments. In the context of osteotomy planning, the CTJ definition can extend to include T2 and T3 [59]. This region also encompasses the thoracic inlet, a stable bony circle formed by the first ribs on both sides, the T1 vertebral body, and the upper part of the sternum. From a biomechanical perspective, the CTJ marks the transition from the highly mobile cervical spine to the relatively rigid thoracic spine. Additionally, it's the point where cervical lordosis transforms into thoracic kyphosis. This curvature shift exerts significant stress on the CTJ, both in static and dynamic conditions [59, 60].

The sagittal alignment of the cranium and cervical spine is influenced by the shape and orientation of the thoracic inlet, crucial for maintaining a balanced, upright posture and horizontal gaze, akin to the relationship between pelvic incidence and lumbar lordosis (LL) [55]. Lee et al. [55] revealed significant associations between the thoracic inlet angle and cranial offset as well as craniocervical alignment. The neck typically tilts at around 45 degrees to minimize the energy expended by neck muscles. This implies that a smaller thoracic inlet angle results in a smaller T1 slope and reduced

Segmental cervical angles [28]		C2-C7 lordosis [31]		
Level	**Angle (deg)**	**Age group**	**Men (deg)**	**Women (deg)**
C0-C1	2.1 ± 5.0	20–25	16 ± 16	15 ± 10
C1-C2	−32.2 ± 7.0	30–35	21 ± 14	16 ± 16
C2-C3	−1.9 ± 5.2	40–45	27 ± 14	23 ± 17
C3-C4	−1.5 ± 5.0	50–55	22 ± 15	25 ± 11
C4-C5	−0.6 ± 4.4	60–65	22 ± 13	25 ± 16
C5-C6	−1.1 ± 5.1			
C6-C7	−4.5 ± 4.3			
C2-C7	−9.6			
total (C1-C7)	−41.8			
cervical sagittal vertical axis [28]				
odontoid marker at C7	15.6 ± 11.2 mm			
odontoid marker at sacrum	13.2 ± 29.5 mm			

[Values presented as the means ± SD and the negative sign indicates lordosis in the segmental values].

Table 1.
Normal cervical spinal values in asymptomatic adults from the literature.

	20–39 years		40–59 years		>60 years		P value
	Mean	**SD**	**Mean**	**SD**	**Mean**	**SD**	
C2-C7 Cervical Lordosis (°)	+9.4	9	+6.6	9	+22.2*	9	<0.001
T4-T12 Thoracic Kyphosis (°)	−38.1	11	−36	9	−45	14	NS
L1-S1 Lumbar Lordosis (°)	+61.5	12	+60.3	7	+55.7	13	NS
Pelvic Tilt (°)	12.1	7	14.5	5	15.1	8	NS
Pelvic Incidence (°)	52.1	10	54.3	8	53.5	10	NS
Sacral Slope (°)	40	9	39.9	7	36.5	10	NS
SVA (mm)	−28.5	28	−18.2	39	22.4*	40	<0.001
T1-Slope (°)	−22	7	−21.1	8	−31.6*	9	0.001

NS = non significant. Adapted from Blondel et al. [56].

Table 2.
Mean sagittal parameters among the volunteers stratified by age group, p-values refer to ANOVA comparison between groups.

cervical lordosis angle to sustain the natural neck tilt, and vice versa. The T1 inclination is instrumental in determining the requisite subaxial lordosis to maintain the head's center of gravity in equilibrium. This value varies depending on global spinal alignment, assessed through SVA, and inherent upper thoracic kyphosis. In cases of scoliosis, the T1 sagittal angle has been shown to directly correlate with SVA, measured from the C2 dens plumb line, offering a measure of overall sagittal alignment [61].

It's important to recognize that the cervical, thoracic, lumbar, and pelvic spinal regions are interrelated, with several significant correlations identified [56]. Blondel et al. [56] explored various spinal parameters in asymptomatic volunteers and observed that pelvic incidence (PI) correlated with LL, LL correlated with thoracic kyphosis (TK), and TK correlated with cervical lordosis (CL). Consequently, an increase in PI corresponded to an increase in LL, which, in turn, correlated with an increase in TK, subsequently influencing CL. However, there was no observed correlation between PI and TK, which adds complexity to the correlation chain from the pelvis to the cervical spine. The prevailing view suggests that LL is proportionate to PI and TK, given that PI is a fixed parameter with limited flexibility. Individuals with a smaller PI or lesser TK exhibited reduced LL compared to those with small PI and more substantial TK. This underscores that TK does not result from LL; instead, LL is a consequence of TK and PI. As mentioned earlier, CL was linked to TK, indicating that as TK increases, so does CL. Nevertheless, this CL adjustment, while substantial, is often insufficient to maintain the head's alignment over the pelvis, though it does suffice to ensure a horizontally oriented gaze. Moreover, CL was found to correlate with SVA, pelvic tilt (PT), and T1 slope. Subjects with a positive SVA displayed increased cervical lordosis, regardless of whether their SVA fell within the normal range of values. This adaptation in cervical lordosis to sagittal global alignment represents a compensatory mechanism aimed at preserving a horizontal gaze, similar to the roles of thoracic kyphosis and lumbar lordosis. When both LL and TK adjust in response to the patient's PI, cervical lordosis aligns proportionately with the other spinal curves. However, when there's an anterior malalignment of the spine due to a loss of lumbar lordosis and/or an increase in thoracic kyphosis, an augmented cervical lordosis serves as a compensatory mechanism.

4. Clinical evaluation of the cervical deformity patient

When evaluating a patient with cervical deformity in the preoperative setting, the primary goal is to determine the ideal amount and type of correction as well as how to achieve this desired correction. As of now, an established optimal postoperative cervical lordosis does not exist, however, a general guideline for correcting any cervical kyphosis is to achieve at least a neutral alignment [62]. In addition to the medical history and physical exam, a comprehensive assessment of the previously mentioned radiographic parameters should be conducted: specifically CL, cSVA, CBVA, and T1S-CL. Understanding these values for a given patient will aid in determining the surgical techniques required to achieve these specific goals. In cervical deformity surgery, there is no gold standard for "normal values" of these parameters, however, the current available evidence suggests that generally accepted targets include cSVA <40 mm, T1S-CL <15°, and CBVA between −10° and + 20° [14, 15, 43, 63–65].

4.1 Medical history and physical exam

The medical history and physical exam is vital to the proper assessment of the adult cervical deformity patient. This will lead to an appropriate evaluation of the preoperative risk as well as the correct deformity classification and subsequently the surgical management. The initial phase of this procedure commences with a comprehensive medical history review and physical examination. The medical history plays a pivotal role, particularly in cases involving high-risk and fragile surgical patients. Consequently, an extensive medical history becomes instrumental in tailoring the treatment approach and facilitating discussions about potential risks. Pertinent aspects include significant medical comorbidities, smoking history, and the utilization of nonsteroidal anti-inflammatory drugs (NSAIDs). Therefore, preoperative medications and social habits should be reviewed thoroughly. Patients suffering from severe cervical deformities that have significant neck pain are many times on chronic opioids. It is thus critical to make every effort to wean off of these medications prior to surgery to help improve the postoperative outcomes and to minimize the risk of narcotic overdose [65]. Furthermore, medications as well as dietary supplements that can result in excessive bleeding such as ginger, gingko, fish oils, aspirin, etc. should all be stopped. Smoking cessation and normalization of vitamin D levels must also be addressed. And finally, the patient's general medical status and medical comorbidities must be carefully evaluated. Due to a significant number of because of complex comorbidities, some patients may not be medically fit for an extensive surgical correction and less invasive procedure or medical management may be needed instead.

The physical exam should start with a complete neurological exam and also include an assessment of the patient standing upright with hips and knees fully extended as well as in the sitting and supine positions [15, 16]. These additional physical exam positions can add a significant amount of insight into the patients' type of cervical deformity. For the sitting position, the effect of any lumbar and/or pelvic/hip deformity on the cervical spine. When the patient is in the supine position, the examiner can assess the rigidity of the deformity under the direct effect of gravity. Depending on the flexibility/rigidity of the deformity, the patients head may or may not be able to lay flat on the exam table. Patients with a fixed primary cervical deformity exhibit enduring cervical flexion even when in a supine position, which is in contrast to individuals with thoracic, lumbar, or hip deformities, as they tend to correct their posture when seated or lying down. Additionally, it is essential to measure CBVA both before and after surgery using the chin-brow to vertical angle method, utilizing clinical photographs of the patient in a standing position with their hips and knees extended, and their neck maintained in a neutral or fixed position. The CBVA measurement assists in determining the extent of posterior osteotomy wedge removal based on the angle, contributing to surgical planning. Patients experiencing head ptosis or neck drop, a condition known as cervical camptocormia, often present with a flexible sagittal spinal deformity that corrects itself when they lie in a supine position. Cervical camptocormia can stem from various causes, including different myopathies, amyotrophic lateral sclerosis (ALS), parkinsonism disorders, and idiopathic factors [66]. Therefore, the initial evaluation of a patient with camptocormia (or any other flexible deformity) should encompass relevant electromyography and nerve conduction studies, coupled with a referral to Neurology to rule out a primary myopathy or ALS. Furthermore, it is advisable to refer these patients to physical therapy before considering surgical correction and fusion as potential treatment options.

4.2 Cervical deformity and myelopathy

If a cervical deformity patient shows signs of myelopathy on the physical exam, this could be from direct spinal cord compression as evidenced on the MRI or from the deformity itself [67]. However it is likely a result of a combination of both and it's important to understand the relationship of cervical deformity and myelopathy. Progressive cervical kyphosis has been associated with myelopathy even without central stenosis [67]. The myelopathy is a consequence of cervical kyphosis, which leads to the sagging of the spinal cord against the vertebral bodies. This sagging results in anterior spinal cord damage and an escalation in the longitudinal tension on the cord due to its tethering by the dentate ligaments and cervical nerve roots [67–69]. As the cervical kyphosis continues to progress over time, the spinal cord undergoes compression, becoming flattened against the posterior aspect of the vertebral bodies. This results in the tethering of the cervical cord, leading to an increase in intramedullary pressure, subsequently causing neuronal loss and cord demyelination [70–72]. Furthermore, the deformity also has a flattening effect on the small blood vessels located on the spinal cord's surface, resulting in reduced blood supply and ischemia [67, 70, 72–74]. Smith and colleagues [75] investigated myelopathy scores via the modified Japanese Orthopedic Association (mJOA) scale with cervical sagittal alignment and spinal cord volume in patients with myelopathy. They found a moderate negative correlation in patients with cervical kyphosis between cord volume and cross sectional area to mJOA scores (i.e., as the kyphosis is larger the cord volume gets smaller). A positive correlation (opposite) was found for patients with cervical lordosis (as the cervical lordosis increases so does the spinal cord volume) thus indicating a relationship of cord volume to myelopathy that differs on the basis of cervical spine sagittal alignment [75]. Therefore sagittal myelopathy in the cervical deformity patient may be largely form the cervical kyphosis and must be considered in the clinical evaluation and preoperative surgical planning.

4.3 Radiographic evaluation

After a comprehensive medical history and physical exam, every patient should have a 36-inch standing plain film x-ray (or EOS scan described below) and dynamic flexion/extension cervical plain x-ray films. The 36-inch standing film (or EOS) allows for cervical alignment measurements in the context of critical global spinal alignment parameters. The flexion/extension xrays aid in determining the relative rigidity of the cervical spine as well as any atlantoaxial instability. With regard to the standing 36 inch x-rays, the EOS system gives single planar standing x-rays from the skull to the feet and allows a 3-dimensional (3D) configuration of the entire spine [76]. The advantages of this system include: (1) the entire body can be imaged at once thus obviating the need for joining multiple separate x-rays, (2) the x-ray images can be re-formatted into 3D configuration, (3) the delivered radiation dose is 1/10th of the standard x-rays (4) all the points of alignment and related compensation throughout the spine, pelvis, and/or lower extremities are imaged simultaneously [77]. Furthermore, studies have shown that the EOS system is highly accurate, reproducible, and precise in the measurement of spinal curvature [78–81]. The x-rays mentioned above proved the radiographic foundation for any cervical deformity patient, however, additional radiographic studies are generally performed which include computed tomography (CT) and magnetic resonance imaging (MRI). The CT scans are used to assess for osseous landmarks to plan for instrumentation insertion, evaluate bone quality, and any prior instrumentation which the MRI can aid in evaluating areas of stenosis resulting in neural compromise and spinal cord tethering. Sometimes a CT scan can help determining the extent of fusion and osteophyte changes at the disc and can be important in decision making to assess the need for osteotomies to correct the deformity.

4.4 Cervical deformity classification

Once the surgeon has a comprehensive assessment of the patient form a medical history, physical exam, and radiographic stand point, the patients' deformity can then be classified to help guide surgical planning. A classification system has recently been proposed by Ames and colleagues [14] whereas until then, there was no comprehensive cervical spine deformity classification system. Not only does this system aid in surgeon planning, but it also provides a mechanism for clear communication among surgeons and places the cervical deformity in the context of global spinal alignment and clinically relevant radiographic parameters as well as myelopathy. The classification system involves a primary deformity descriptor that describes the location of the apex as five different modifiers (**Table 3**). The modifiers include radiographically measured parameters and a clinical score for the degree of myelopathy per the mJOA scale. All of the five modifiers used in this classification had been previously shown to have a clinical impact [14].

The classification system commences by using a deformity descriptor to establish a fundamental categorization of various deformity types and their respective locations. The initial three types pertain to primary sagittal deformities, distinguishing them based on the deformity apex's position. Type C corresponds to cases where the curve apex is situated in the cervical spine, Type CT denotes instances with the apex at the cervico-thoracic junction, and Type T designates those with the apex located in the thoracic spine. Primary coronal deformities are defined as those exhibiting a C2-C7 coronal Cobb angle exceeding 15°, and they are denoted as Type S. As for the remaining deformity types occurring at the cranio-vertebral junction, they are categorized under Type CVJ.

Among the five modifiers present in the classification system, three pertain to sagittal alignment parameters. These include cSVA, horizontal gaze (assessed through CBVA), and the variance between cervical lordosis and the T1 slope (CL-T1S). Each of these parameters was specifically chosen due to its direct correlation with patients' HRQOL14, and they are each divided into three distinct severity grades, as indicated in **Table 3**. The inclusion of cSVA is justified by the substantial influence of sagittal alignment on HRQOL in patients with thoracolumbar spinal deformities, supported by studies like those conducted by of Tang et al. [54]. and Smith et al. [75], which establish the connection between cervical sagittal alignment and HRQOL. CBVA is integrated into the system because horizontal gaze holds a fundamental significance in basic human functioning, with previous research underscoring the importance of accounting for horizontal gaze in spine deformity surgery [15, 43–48, 82]. Furthermore, the connection between the T1 slope and cervical lordosis can be likened to the relationship between pelvic incidence (PI) and lumbar lordosis (LL) in the lower back. Just as a higher T1 slope necessitates a more substantial degree of cervical lordosis to align the head properly over the thoracic inlet and trunk, a greater PI demands a greater degree of lumbar lordosis to achieve balance in the lumbar spine [15, 53]. And moreover, since cervical kyphosis is the most common type of cervical deformity having a large clinical impact, a classification parameter reflective of cervical lordosis is included as a modifier for the classification.

The last two modifiers pertain to myelopathy and the overall spinal alignment, as defined by the SRS-Schwab thoracolumbar deformity classification. As previously mentioned, understanding the relationship between myelopathy and cervical alignment is pivotal when assessing patients with cervical deformities. The presence of myelopathy can significantly influence the surgical approach, as it necessitates addressing spinal cord compromise when it is present. This can be accomplished through direct decompression, deformity correction, or a combination of both interventions. Consequently, the classification system includes a measure of myelopathy, employing the mJOA score, which is a widely recognized and accepted quantitative

Deformity Descriptor
C: Primary sagittal deformity apex in the cervical spine
CT: Primary sagittal deformity apex at the cervico-thoracic junction
T: Primary sagittal deformity apex in the thoracic spine
S: Primary coronal deformity
CVJ: primary cranio-vertebral junction deformity
5 Modifiers
C2-C7 sagittal vertical axis
0: C2-C7 SVA <4 cm
1: C2-C7 SVA <4 cm to 8 cm
2: C2-C7 SVA >8 cm
Horizontal gaze
0: CBVA 1°-10°
1: CBVA −10° to 0°
2: CBVA <-10° to >25°
Cervical lordosis minus T1 slope
0: CL-T1 < 15°
1: CL-T1 15° to 20°
2: CL-T1 > 20°
Myelopathy
0: mJOA = 18 (None)
1: mJOA = 15–17 (Mild)
2: mJOA = 12–14 (Moderate)
3: mJOA = <12 (Severe)
SRS-Schwab Classification
T, L, D, or N: Curve type
0, +, or ++: PI-LL grades
0, +, or ++: Pelvic tilt grades
0, +, or ++: C7-S1 SVA grades

CBVA = chin brow vertical angle, CL = cervical lordosis, mJOA = modified Japanese Orthopedic Association, T = thoracic, L = lordosis, D = double, N = none, LL = lumbar lordosis, PI = pelvic incidence. SRS = Scoliosis Research Society.

Table 3.
Cervical deformity classification system by Ames et al. [14].

assessment of spondylotic myelopathy severity. The scores on this scale range from 0 to 18, with lower scores indicating a more severe impact from myelopathy. As a result, three distinct groups of scores with increasing severity were integrated into the classification system (**Table 3**).

Lastly, the incorporation of global spinal alignment through the SRS-Schwab classification was deemed essential because spinal segments do not operate in isolation. Cervical deformities can influence thoracolumbar deformities, and conversely, thoracolumbar deformities may generate or contribute to cervical deformities [15]. This interdependence is underscored by Smith et al's findings, which reveal that adults with positive sagittal spinopelvic malalignment adjust by increasing cervical lordosis to maintain a horizontal gaze. Moreover, surgical correction of thoracolumbar sagittal malalignment leads to the amelioration of abnormal cervical hyperlordosis through reciprocal adjustments [83]. Ha and colleagues subsequently corroborated this observation, pinpointing key radiographic parameters associated with these compensatory alterations [84]. Furthermore, there is a notable prevalence of concomitant cervical deformities among adults with thoracolumbar deformities [85]. As a result, it became evident that the assessment and classification of cervical deformities should not be conducted in isolation. Instead, it is imperative to consider the alignment of the thoracolumbar spine and pelvis. Consequently, the SRS-Schwab classification for adult thoracolumbar spinal deformities was integrated as a modifier within the cervical deformity classification (**Table 1**). The validity of the SRS-Schwab classification has been established, showcasing its correlation with HRQOL measures at the outset and its sensitivity to changes in disease state [49, 86, 87].

5. Surgical planning

Following a thorough examination that encompasses a detailed medical history, an extensive neurological evaluation, and a comprehensive physical assessment, as well as the necessary imaging and radiographic measurements, and the categorization of the deformity, the groundwork for preoperative surgical planning can commence if the patient is deemed suitable for surgery. The key considerations for surgical planning encompass the following factors:

1. The evaluation of neural compression and any accompanying neurological symptoms.

2. The determination of deformity flexibility or rigidity.

3. Assessment of anterior or posterior ankylosis.

4. Examination of the location of the deformity.

5. Review of any previous cervical spine surgeries.

6. Inspection for degenerative changes at other spinal levels, notably the proximal and distal vertebral levels and the cervicothoracic junction.

7. Evaluation of the patient's overall medical condition and the presence of any relevant medical comorbidities, as previously mentioned [65].

Some surgeons have advocated cervical traction pre-operatively to facilitate deformity correction prior to surgery. In most cases, a period of 3 to 5 days under traction is typically adequate for achieving a reduction in the deformity [62]. In the event of a successful reduction of the cervical deformity, posterior only fixation and fusion techniques may be adequate to treat the deformity.

In general, anterior approach enables better and more harmonious correction of deformities through interbody release and instrumentation that leverages both biomechanical principles and posture adjustment to achieve the desired postoperative cervical alignment. Any ventral compression of the spinal cord should also be noted on the MRI. If anterior compression is present, then a ventral approach may be necessary in the overall strategy in order to achieve anterior spinal cord decompression [15, 65]. In the setting of infection or neoplasm, if the integrity of the anterior column is compromised, then the anterior approach is preferred to establish anterior column support [65].

The assessment of cervical spine flexibility and rigidity plays a pivotal role in determining the appropriate surgical course, as discussed previously. When clinical examination, dynamic x-rays, and CT scans confirm the cervical spine's flexibility and absence of ankylosis, either an anterior or posterior correction approach can be considered.

For many flexible deformities, a posterior-only correction method might be applicable. However, in cases of severe kyphotic deformities, relying solely on a posterior approach might prove insufficient to rectify the deformity, necessitating an additional anterior approach. In situations where the deformity is identified as rigid, it is advisable to obtain a high-resolution CT scan of the cervical spine to assess the presence of anterior and posterior ankyloses. If the spine exhibits rigidity without ankylosed facets or has a history of prior instrumentation, employing an anterior-only approach may suffice, but if anterior fusion is more than three levels, posterior fixation should be considered to minimize risk of pseudarthrosis [65].

When the anterior column of the spine is rigid and features ankylosed facets, a combination of both anterior and posterior strategies may be employed to address the deformity. In such instances, either a 360- or 540-degree approach may be utilized to achieve circumferential release and deformity correction. The exact choice may depend on the specific deformity and surgeon's training and preference.

In the senior author's experience, anterior release and interbody fusion followed by posterior osteotomy and fixation is typically adequate to treat even circumferentially ankylosed cervical deformities. Some surgeons may prefer to initiate the correction process with a posterior release, followed by anterior release and fusion, and then followed by posterior fixation. This posterior-anterior-posterior, or 540-degree approach can be useful in revision cases where posterior instrumentation is present.

The precise location of the kyphotic deformity holds significant importance, influencing the choice of approach, type of osteotomy, and correction strategy for the specific cervical deformity under treatment. In general, when dealing with focal cervical sagittal plane deformities in the subaxial region (referred to as cervical kyphosis), a combination of anterior release and posterior fixation frequently yields the most effective results.

For patients presenting with cervical deformities arising from issues at the cervicothoracic junction (characterized by a high T1-slope, neutral to normal cervical lordosis, and a high low C2-slope), the appropriate strategy typically involves a three-column osteotomy in cervicothoracic junction with a posterior approach.

In situations where cervical deformity coexists with severe thoracic kyphosis, additional osteotomies in the thoracic spine may be necessary to achieve the desired correction in the cervical region. Notably, increased kyphosis in the upper thoracic region can negatively impact the T1S (T1 slope), and a comprehensive correction of T1S and cSVA (cranial sagittal vertical axis) may necessitate a significant surgical intervention extending into the mid-thoracic level [65].

Nonetheless, this approach remains a subject of controversy, and additional data is needed to substantiate the viability of such assertive surgical methods. However, as a general guideline, when patients necessitate deformity correction above the T2 level and concurrently present with lower thoracic deformities, it is advisable to address the lower deformity initially. In cases where the reverse sequence is pursued, rectifying the cervical deformity first to achieve a horizontal gaze might subsequently result in an overcorrected positioning of the head and neck when addressing the lower thoracic deformity [65].

Coronal cervical deformities can occur independently or in conjunction with sagittal deformities, often exhibiting a range of severity levels, which are collectively referred to as fixed multiplanar deformities. Patients presenting with such deformities may necessitate the implementation of three-column osteotomies to rectify the spinal alignment in both the coronal and sagittal planes, as well as to alleviate pressure on the spinal cord and nerves [15]. Furthermore, a multifaceted approach involving multiple stages might be imperative. This could entail the adoption of a 540-degree circumferential osteotomy or even a cervical vertebral column resection (VCR) [88–90].

Lastly, in the case of patients with a history of previous cervical spine fusion, it is of paramount importance, to ensure the surgery's safety and smooth execution, to acquire the operative report. This report is instrumental in identifying the specific instrumentation employed during the prior procedure, as well as any intraoperative discoveries. Additionally, a comprehensive evaluation of the previous fusion mass should be conducted using CT scans to assess the presence of any pseudarthrosis. If an anterior approach was done previously, it may be preferable to enter the contralateral side for the planned upcoming surgery as prior scar tissues may make the tissue dissection much more difficult [65]. An otolaryngology consultation may be obtained preoperatively to confirm vocal cord motility bilaterally if planning on entering the contralateral side. Should injury to the recurrent or superior laryngeal nerve occur or if, for any reason, an evaluation by Otolaryngology is needed, it is imperative to err on the side of caution by opting for the same side to minimize the risk of potential bilateral damage to the laryngeal nerves [65]. Depending on ones' comfort level and the institution, the Otolaryngology colleagues may assist in exposure to help minimize risk to the nerves and surrounding structures given the amount of scar tissue. In the event that a prior posterior approach was undertaken, it becomes imperative to examine the surgical site meticulously for the integrity of the surrounding soft tissues. If any observation reveals the separation or detachment of the posterior paraspinal muscles, or if a significant void within the wound or inadequate soft tissue coverage is identified, the risk of potential complications related to the wound increases. In such cases, it becomes necessary to mobilize and reattach any detached muscles from their lateral positions back to the midline. If the surgeon lacks experience in these specialized techniques, it is advisable to seek a consultation with a plastic surgeon who can provide expertise in managing the complexities of wound closure [65].

6. Surgical techniques

Cervical deformity surgery has multiple goals and includes the correction of deformity, re-establishment of horizontal gaze, stabilization of the cervical spine, and decompression of the neural elements. The choice of surgical technique for

DOI: http://dx.doi.org/10.5772/intechopen.1003591

correction involves a careful assessment of the patient including a history and physical, neurologic examination, and evaluation of radiographic data. Careful surgical technique is critical to decreasing the risk of complications related to cervical spine deformity correction. Methods to correct cervical spine deformity include anterior-only, posterior-only, and a combination of anterior and posterior approaches. In this paper, surgical techniques including anterior and posterior techniques are discussed.

6.1 Anterior surgical techniques

6.1.1 Anterior cervical discectomy and fusion

Anterior cervical discectomy and fusion (ACDF) is perhaps one of the most familiar procedures to spine surgeons. The use of ACDF allows the sequential induction of lordosis via distraction over multiple segments. Furthermore, additional lordosis can be induced via sequential screw tightening, which pulls the spine towards a lordotic cervical plate [91]. A single level ACDF may increase the overall C2-C7 lordosis by 3.5 degrees after 1 year [92]. If the patient has had prior ventral cervical spine surgery, vocal cord function should be assessed by otolaryngologists prior to performing another anterior surgery to determine the approach to the cervical spine. If there is no history of prior injury, then the authors of this paper approach the cervical from the left side to reduce the risk of injury to the recurrent laryngeal nerve, which has a longer course on the left side. If the patient is shown to have prior vocal cord function impairment, then the approach should be performed from the ipsilateral side as prior surgery to avoid placing the contralateral vocal cord at risk.

The patient is placed under general endotracheal anesthesia and maintained in the supine position. Bumps may be placed under the shoulders to encourage extension of the head but care must be taken to ensure that the head is not floating. The traditional approach to the anterior cervical spine is well described via the Smith-Robinson approach [93]. The incision can be performed utilizing either a transverse or longitudinal incision. During this approach, the omohyoid muscle is identified and divided by monopolar cautery. If the superior and inferior thyroid arteries are encountered, they may be ligated and divided to maximize the surgical exposure. However, if the superior thyroid artery is encountered, then it should be separated from adjacent structures to prevent injury to the superior laryngeal nerve, a portion of which often accompanies the superior laryngeal artery. The trachea and esophagus are mobilized carefully, and the longus colli muscles are released with bipolar cautery. A table-mounted retractor system is utilized to provide retraction of one disc space at a time.

Once the disc space is identified using lateral fluoroscopy, the anterior osteophytes are first removed using combination of Leksell rongeur and high-speed burr. Subsequent to this, Caspar pins are placed in the vertebral bodies above and below the disc space along with a retractor to distract the disc space. The anterior longitudinal ligament and disc annulus are incised and the disc material is removed utilizing a combination of curettes, pituitary rongeurs, and high-speed burr. The posterior osteophytes should be removed utilizing a high-speed burr and the posterior portion of the uncinate processes. The PLL is identified by looking for fibers traversing in a rostral-caudal direction and removed using small curettes and Kerrison rongeurs.

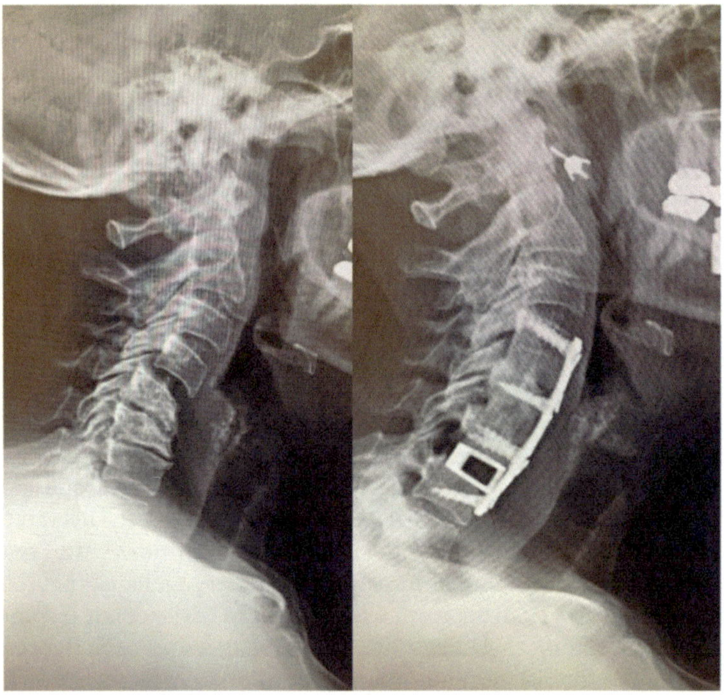

Figure 5.
Cervical deformity correction via anterior only approach with anterior plating.

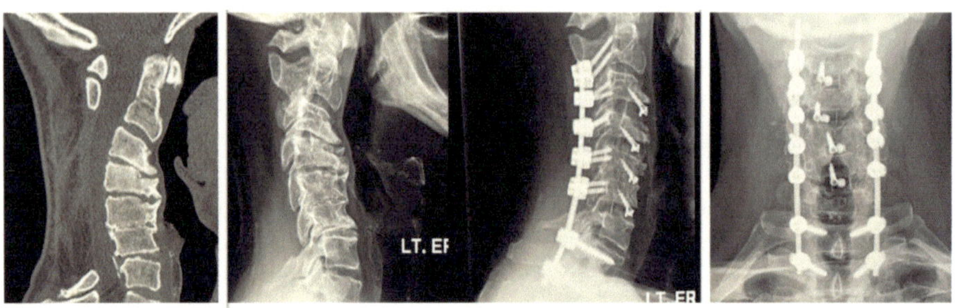

Figure 6.
Cervical deformity correction via combined anterior-posterior approach with standalone cages in front with additional posterior instrumentation.

Mechanical correction of kyphotic deformity can be achieved by utilization sequentially disc spacers in combination with intervertebral body spreaders. The graft with autograft/allograft is subsequently placed into the disc space with sequential lateral fluoroscopic guidance to confirm placement. This process is repeated for each disc level. If an anterior only procedure is performed, then the authors prefer utilizing anterior plates (**Figure 5**). If the surgery involves a posterior fixation in addition, then standalone cages may be used (**Figure 6**).

Additional deformity correction may be achieved by utilizing a long anterior cervical plate which is first fixed into place with screws at the apex of the deformity followed by sequential placement and tightening of screws further and further away from the apex to "pull" the spine towards the lordotic cervical plate [91].

6.1.2 Anterior cervical corpectomy and fusion

The approach for an anterior cervical corpectomy is the same as an ACDF. An anterior cervical discectomy is performed above and below the intended corpectomy level. A Leksell rongeur is utilized to remove the vertebral body up to the posterior portion of the vertebral body, which is removed with a high-speed burr. The remaining PLL is subsequently resected.

There are several choices for graft into the corpectomy site, which include iliac crest, fibula, or a cage. It is critical to ensure that the graft is not so deep as to impinge into the spinal canal. An anterior cervical plate, similar to that in an ACDF, should be placed to prevent cage/graft migration (**Figure 7**). It is important to note that anterior cervical corpectomy performed at more than 2 levels has a very high pseudarthrosis rate and therefore posterior fixation should be performed in these situations [94, 95]. The patient should be immobilized in a hard cervical collar for 4–6 weeks to encourage fusion.

6.1.3 Anterior cervical osteotomy

The usage of anterior osteotomy in the cervical spine, performed through an anteriorly fused spine to the level of the transverse foramen bilaterally can be a powerful correction technique applicable throughout the cervical spine. Symmetric anterior osteotomies can be used to "chin-on-chest" deformities while asymmetric anterior osteotomies can assist with "ear-on-shoulder" deformities [96]. This technique has been described by Kim et al. [97]. The patient undergoes general endotracheal anesthesia in the supine position, with bumps placed under the shoulders to suspend the head which is subsequently supported by a foam donut placed on sheets. Traction utilizing Gardner Wells tongues of a chin strap may assist with intubation and allow easier initial approach to the cervical spine.

The choice of laterality for exposure should be determined as described above under the ACDF technique with utilization of preoperative vocal cord examination as necessary. If there is a "ear-on-chest" deformity of significant coronal deformity, it may be easier to approach the spine from the convex side. Dissection is carried out

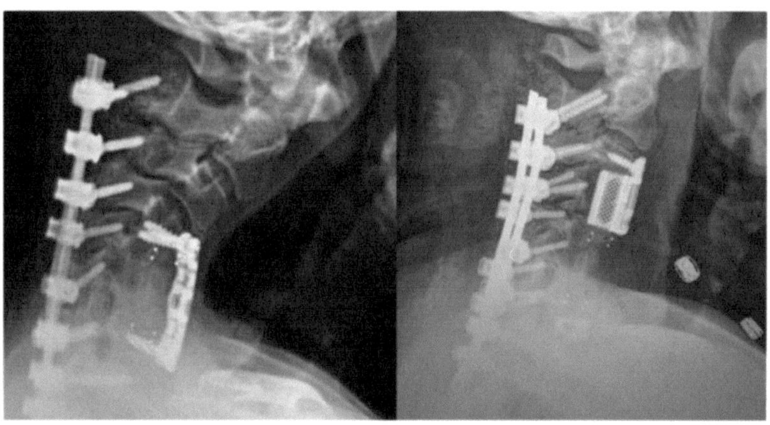

Figure 7.
Cervical deformity correction via anterior corpectomy at C4 with revision posterior spinal instrumentation and fusion.

according to the Smith-Robinson approach. Once the disc level of intended anterior osteotomy is identified, Caspar pins may be placed, perpendicular to the anterior cervical spine to induce lordosis when distraction is performed using the Caspar pin retractor.

Using a high-speed burr, bony resection is started. If there is only kyphotic deformity, then the osteotomy should be performed in a symmetric fashion to avoid inducing coronal deformity. If there is coronal deformity, then an asymmetric resection of bone may facilitate correction of coronal deformity. This bony resection should be performed all the way back to the PLL. As the resection nears the lateral uncinates, the vertebral artery is at risk of injury, and thus a Penfield #2 dissector should be placed at the lateral border of the uncinates to protect the vertebral artery. Once the bone of the lateral uncinate is "egg-shelled" the remainder of the resection should be performed with a microcurette.

Once the osteotomy is performed, the correction of deformity occurs as the surgeon pushes gently on the forehead through the drape. At the same time, sheets may be removed under the head and distraction on the Caspar pins performed to induce lordosis. Other methods to induce lordosis include placement of a Cobb elevator into the osteotomy site with rotation or usage of vertebral body spreaders with sequentially larger disc spacers.

Deformity correction is complete if the occiput touches the operating room table, but if inadequate, the shoulders may be bumped to provide further lordosis and the cervical traction via Chin strap or Gardner Wells tongs may be increased to 25 lb. If there was complete deformity correction, then an anterior cervical plate with fixed angle screws are placed but if there is incomplete correction, then a trapezoidal graft in the anterior portion of the osteotomy site without cervical plate is performed so that further lordosis induction can be performed via a posterior operation (**Figure 8**). It is important to place a buttress plate or an interference screw in this situation however, to prevent the graft from being extruded anteriorly during the posterior portion. Posterior augmentation is recommended for anterior osteotomies, as the endplates are trabecular in nature and at high risk of subsidence. Patients are almost always placed in a hard cervical collar for immobilization for 4–6 weeks to encourage fusion.

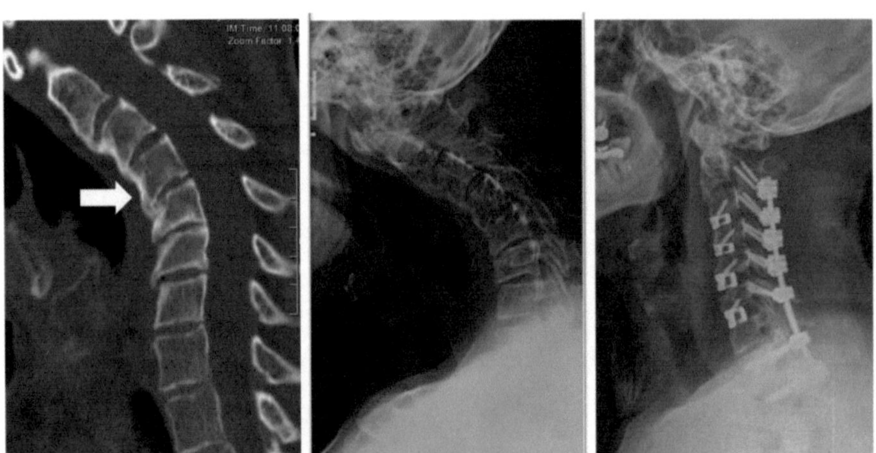

Figure 8.
Cervical deformity correction of a rigid deformity using anterior osteotomies to release fused levels with posterior spinal release, instrumentation and fusion.

6.2 Posterior surgical techniques

6.2.1 Posterior instrumentation and fusion with or without decompression

Patients who have a deformity curve which is flexible without a significant source of ventral compression may benefit from a posterior-only instrumentation and fusion. This procedure is quite commonly performed among spine surgeons.

The patient undergoes general endotracheal anesthesia. Subsequently, pinning for fixation of the head occurs, either utilizing a Mayfield head holder and system or Gardner-Wells tongs with a bivector setup utilizing two separate ropes at different angles to stabilize the neck prior to instrumentation, and another rope to induce extension after osteotomy/correction with 15–20 lb. of weight on the rope. After pinning, the patient is flipped prone and the table is subsequently placed in a reverse Trendelenburg position.

A midline incision is performed with meticulous division into the midline raphe. Careful subperiosteal exposure of the laminae and lateral masses are performed to minimize blood loss. At C2 there are a variety of options for instrumentation, including the placement of pars screws, pedicle screws, or translaminar screws. From C3-C6 typically lateral mass screws are placed, and at C7 there is an option for either lateral mass of pedicle screw fixation, although typically if fixation is extended into the upper thoracic spine, C7 is skipped to allow space for screw fixation of T1. At T1 and T2, pedicle screw fixation is utilization.

Decompression via laminectomy can be performed either before or after placement of screws, although the placement of rods and deformity correction itself usually takes place after the laminectomies are performed. Arthrodesis is performed after copious irrigation of the surgical cavity via thorough decortication and subsequent bone graft placement. Vancomycin powder may be used to decrease the chance of infection. One or more deep subfascial drains are placed. Occasionally, a more superficial subdermal drain may be added if the wound is particularly deep with excess adipose tissue.

During closure, muscles are reapproximated and multi-layer closure is performed with interrupted sutures.

6.2.2 Smith-Peterson osteotomy

Smith-Peterson Osteotomies (SPOs) also known as "Ponte Osteotomy" when performed at multiple levels, are performed as part of a posterior instrumentation and fusion with or without decompression. The SPO is performed by completely resecting the superior articulating facet, inferior articulating facet at a joint, along with removing the ligamentum flavum, lamina, and spinous processes (**Figure 9**). It is important that there is residual anterior column mobility to obtain correction of kyphotic deformity during this osteotomy. After the SPO is performed, compression of the posterior elements is performed with rod and screw fixation to close the osteotomy. Risks of SPO include compression of nerve roots as the osteotomy is closed due to compression from pedicles or residual superior articulating facets.

6.2.3 Pedicle subtraction osteotomy

When there is severe, fixed cervical kyphotic deformity the cervical pedicle subtraction osteotomy may be the preferred technique for deformity correction. The

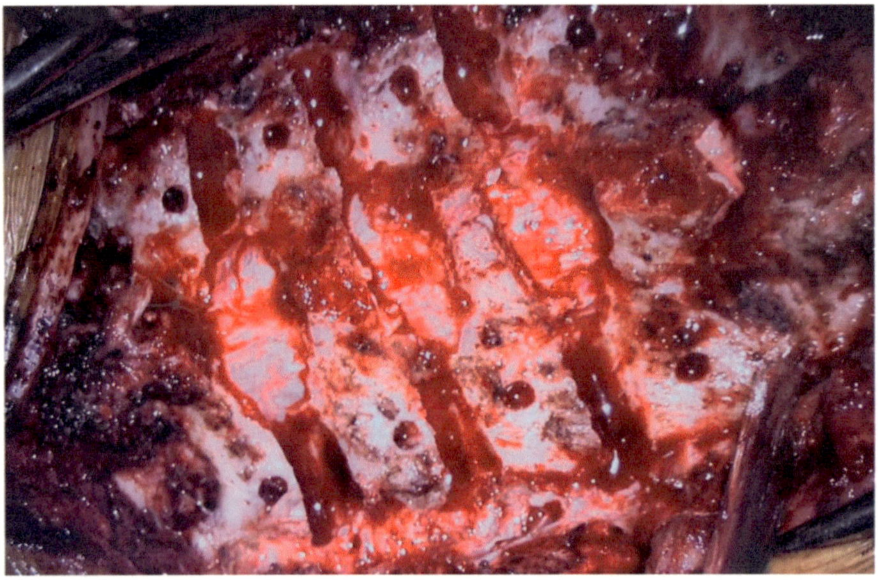

Figure 9.
Cervical Smith-Petersen osteotomies for posterior release of a rigid deformity.

patient is induced with general endotracheal anesthesia and flipped into the prone position after fixation with Mayfield or Gardner Wells tongs as previously described. As described previously, the Gardner Wells tongs are used with two ropes, which allows extension for osteotomy closure after the pedicle subtraction osteotomy is performed. If a Mayfield clamp is utilized, then the clamp should be released and the head should be placed in a gently extended position to close the osteotomy.

Ideally, the PSO is performed at the cervicothoracic junction for several different reasons. At the cervicothoracic junction, the vertebral artery is further away, the spinal cord is more mobile due to the larger size of the canal, and a C8 nerve root injury is typically less debilitating for hand function. However, it is important to assess the vascular course of the vertebral artery as there can be aberrant courses of vertebral arteries which transverse the C7 transverse foramen.

Exposure and instrumentation of the cervical spine is placed as described above for posterior instrumentation and fusion. Subsequent to this, a C7 laminectomy is performed along with the caudal C6 lamina and the cranial T1 lamina. Utilizing high-speed burr and Leksell rongeur, the C7 lateral masses are removed along with the caudal aspect of C6 inferior facet and the cranial aspect of the T1 superior facet. The pedicles of T1 are fully exposed to ensure there is no superior articular process cranial to the T1 pedicle that remains as this can cause injury to the C8 nerve root during osteotomy closure. The C7 and C8 nerve roots should be visualized.

The thecal sac and C7/C8 nerve roots are protected with cottonoid patties and the cancellous bone of the C7 pedicle is drilled out with burr while leaving the cortical walls intact. The burr should be passed deeper into the body of C7 to remove the cancellous bone of the C7 body. The cortical rim of the C7 pedicles is subsequently removed with small pituitary rongeur and small reverse-angle curettes. The entire pedicle should be removed to avoid compression of nerve roots during osteotomy closure. Utilizing small round tamps and reverse angled curettes, a cavity is formed within the posterior superior portion of the vertebral body and the bone is subsequently pushed anterior into this cavity. Following this, the cortical posterior vertebral wall should be pushed into the cavity using Woodson and angled dural elevators.

Rods are then placed into the thoracic pedicle screws and the osteotomy closure performed by extension of the neck. If the Gardner-Wells tongs have been used, then this is performed by pulling on the tongs through the drape while the traction weight is switched by assistant to the extension rope. It is important to examine and C7 and C8 nerve roots during this closure to make sure there is no compression. If there is compression, additional resection of the inferior portion of C6 facet and superior aspect of T1 facet may be needed. The rod is than engaged into the cervical lateral mass and C2 pars/pedicle screws superior to the osteotomy and fixed into the screws with locking caps.

Upper thoracic PSO or VCRs can be a good alternative for C7 PSO for many patients as it poses less danger for hand function and can offer powerful deformity correction (**Figure 10**).

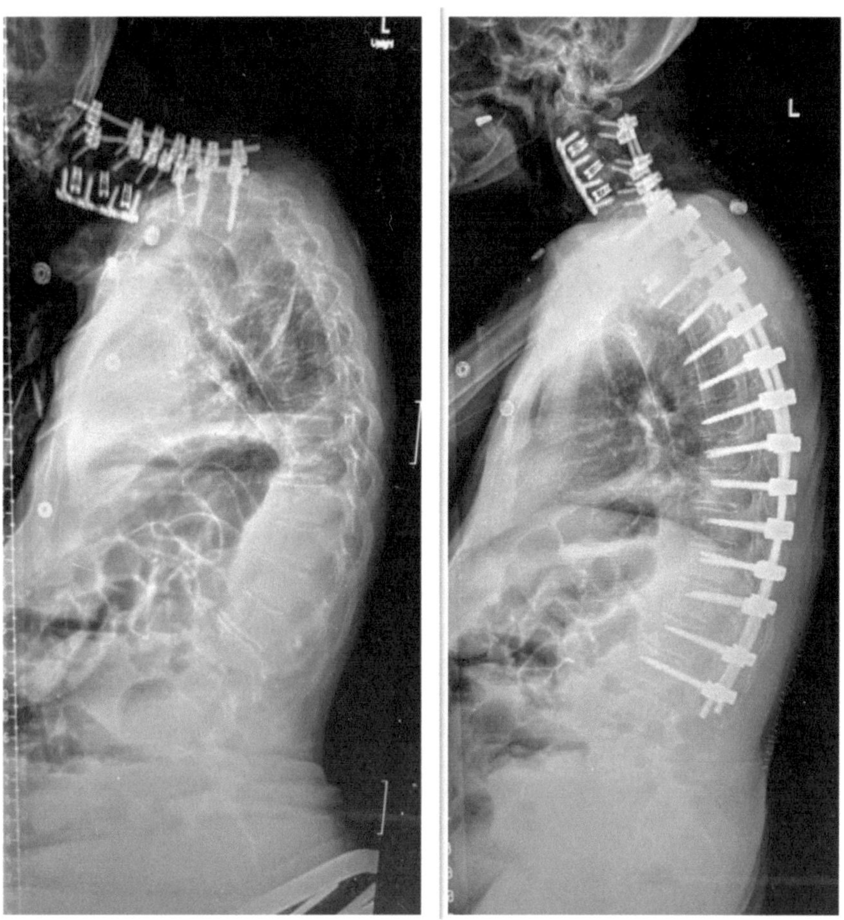

Figure 10.
"Chin-on-chest" deformity due to DJK corrected via posterior only approach by performing a T2 VCR.

Confirmation of correction is performed with lateral X-rays. Arthrodesis is performed with autograft and allograft as described above with careful decortication. Careful multilayer closure is performed along with placement of one or more subfascial drains. The patient should remain in a hard cervical collar for 4–6 weeks after surgery to encourage fusion.

7. Clinical outcome and complication avoidance and future directions

7.1 Clinical outcomes

Clinical outcomes after cervical deformity correction include the physical correction of the kyphosis and the functional outcome of the patient.

7.1.1 Radiographic outcome

In terms of kyphosis correction, the most used measure of horizontal gaze utilized within studies is the Chin-Brow Vertical (CBV) angle, which is determined from photographs. The CBV angle measure the angle between the vertical axis of a patient that is standing upright and a line from the chin to the brow. In severe chin-on-chest type of cervical deformity, this CBV angle may even approach 90 degrees. Multiple studies support a good outcome of kyphosis correction. Simmons and colleagues found that CBV angle improved from 56 degrees to 4 degrees in 114 patients treated with smaller osteotomy and from 49 degrees to 12 degrees in a smaller subset of 17 patients treated with a wider osteotomy, all from a posterior approach [98]. Likewise, Langeloo et al. reported in a group of 16 patients treated via posterior-only approach that CBV angle improved from 42 degrees to 5 degrees resulting in restoration of horizontal gaze in all patients [99]. Tokala et al. found similar results with the posterior approach also, specifically a C7 closing wedge osteotomy technique, with CBV angle improving from 41 degrees to 6 degrees in a group of 8 patients [100].

Another measurement of deformity correction commonly utilized in the literature is the Ishihara index, which is measured on a lateral X-ray. A vertical line is drawn between the posterior-inferior edges of C2 and C7. The perpendicular distances from the line to the posterior-inferior edges of C3, C4, C5, and C6 are summed up and divided by the length of A and multiplied by 100 to determine the Ishihara index. One study by Mummaneni et al. shows that the average Ishihara index improved from a pre-operative value of −17.7 (indicated kyphosis) to +11.4 (indicating lordosis) [101]. This study included 30 patients with cervical kyphotic deformity who underwent circumferential (anterior-posterior combined) spine surgery. Likewise, a review of the literature indicates that there is significant correction of kyphosis as measured by the Cobb angle. Mean correction of kyphosis ranged from 11 to 32 degrees for the anterior only approach, 23.3 degrees to 54 degrees for a posterior only approach, and 24 to 61.3 degrees in a combined anterior-posterior approach in a review of the literature by Etame et al. in 2010 [102]. Radiographically then, cervical deformity surgery appears to result in good outcomes in terms of kyphotic angle correction and CBV angle.

7.1.2 Functional outcomes

Prior studies on cervical deformity correction have measured different functional outcomes after deformity correction. Outcomes measured in prior studies include horizontal gaze, measures of myelopathy (Nurick grade, modified Japanese Orthopedic Association score), measures of spinal cord injury (Frankel grade), and neck pain.

Generally, cervical deformity surgery has excellent outcomes with respect to restoration of horizontal gaze with almost all studies reporting good restoration of horizontal gaze with correction [64, 98, 99, 103, 104].

8. Complications

Surgical correction of cervical spinal deformity is technically challenging as discussed in part 3 and is associated with a high complication rate [105, 106]. A study by Passias and colleagues evaluating a prospective cervical deformity database found a 39.9% intraoperative complication rate [105]. The authors further categorized the complications into various types revealing that the rate of neurological complications stood at 13.9%. Meanwhile, the rates of dysphagia and respiratory issues were 9.8 and 8.2%, respectively. The infections accounted for 8.2%, and the dural tears were documented at 4.1% [105]. In a similar investigation by Smith et al. [106], the comprehensive complication rate in cervical deformity surgery was reported at 43.6%. Among the most frequently encountered complications were dysphagia (11.5%), deep wound infections (6.4%), new C5 palsy (6.4%), and respiratory failures (5.1%).

Smith and colleagues performed another investigation into focusing on all-cause mortality following surgical correction and demonstrated that at 1.2 yrs. postop the all-cause mortality was 9.2%. It goes without saying that the reported rates listed above are high and it is critical to discuss these potential risks and rates of undergoing a surgery for cervical deformity with the patient and to devise an appropriate surgical plan. The complication rate increases in patients undergoing a 3-comumn osteotomy for cervical deformity correction. Smith and colleagues again studied this population and discovered an overall complication rate of 56.5% with neurological deficits being the most common at 17.4% [107]. Among the various surgical procedures, the occurrence of C5 palsy was most frequent when utilizing SPOs, while C8 palsy predominated in cases involving 3-column osteotomies [107].

Postoperative distal junctional kyphosis (DJK) is another critical complication that must be addressed [108, 109]. DJK is typically characterized by a deviation from the expected radiographic alignment, occurring either at one or two levels below the lower-most instrumented vertebra (LIV). This condition has been linked to a range of factors, including adjacent level problems, fixation issues, spondylolisthesis, and various other causes [109]. Passias and colleagues have showed that DJK can occur at a rate of 23.1% 1 year following the cervical deformity correction [109]. The authors showed that DJK is likely to occur at 3 months after the surgery. Furthermore, the patients suffering from DJK were more likely to have severe cervical deformity at baseline [109].

Given the notable prevalence of DJK (Distal Junctional Kyphosis), proactive measures are frequently taken to mitigate its occurrence. These preventive strategies encompass the administration of bone-strengthening medications like teriparatide, the meticulous selection of the Lower Instrumented Vertebra (LIV) with respect to the curvature apex, and the implementation of ligament reinforcement [110]. Furthermore, the positioning of the LIV in relation to the curvature apex plays a pivotal role in DJK prevention. When certain criteria are met, such as a cSVA (cranial sagittal vertical axis) exceeding 4 cm, a T1 slope surpassing 30 degrees, or a global SVA exceeding 8 cm, as well as in cases where patients undergo a 3-column osteotomy, it is imperative for the LIV to be situated below the thoracic apex, typically at T9 or T10. In situations meeting these criteria, the risk of DJK escalates if the LIV is positioned near or above the thoracic apex [111]. Many different considerations must be taking into account for preoperative surgical planning and any possible attempt to reduce potential risks to the patient should be pursued given the high complication rate associated with these surgeries. With the recent expansion of large datasets and complex computation methods, future directions of risk stratification and reduction include predictive models and artificial intelligence that may augment surgical planning and aid in shared surgical decision making with the patients.

9. Conclusion

Cervical deformity correction can be challenging. Goals of cervical deformity surgery include correction of cervical spine deformity to maintain horizontal gaze, decompress neural elements, and restore alignment of the cervical spine. Cervical spine deformity correction can involve several anterior and posterior techniques such as ACDF, anterior osteotomy, posterior instrumentation and arthrodesis, and posterior osteotomies. Careful surgical planning and surgical technique are essential to minimize the risk of complication and maximize clinical outcomes in cervical deformity correction.

Author details

Weiye Zhang[1,2], Wei Tan[3], Samer G. Zammar[2], Kathryn Park[2], Justin Scheer[2], Young Lee[2], Alysha Jamison[2] and Lee A. Tan[2*]

1 Wangjing Hospital, China Academy of Chinese Medical Sciences, Beijing, China

2 Department of Neurological Surgery, University of California, San Francisco, USA

3 The Affiliated Hospital of Guizhou Medical University, Guiyang, China

*Address all correspondence to: lee.tan@ucsf.edu

References

[1] Ailon T, Smith JS, Shaffrey CI, et al. Outcomes of operative treatment for adult cervical deformity: A prospective multicenter assessment with 1-year follow-up. Neurosurgery. 2018;**83**(5):1031-1039

[2] Iyer S, Kim HJ, Bao H, et al. Cervical deformity patients have baseline swallowing dysfunction but surgery does not increase dysphagia at 3 months: Results from a prospective cohort study. Global Spine Journal. 2019;**9**(5):532-539

[3] Miller EK, Ailon T, Neuman BJ, et al. Assessment of a novel adult cervical deformity frailty index as a component of preoperative risk stratification. World Neurosurgery. 2018;**109**:e800-e806

[4] Smith JS, Line B, Bess S, et al. The health impact of adult cervical deformity in patients presenting for surgical treatment: Comparison to United States population norms and chronic disease states based on the EuroQuol-5 dimensions questionnaire. Neurosurgery. 2017;**80**(5):716-725

[5] Smith JS, Shaffrey CI, Kim HJ, et al. Comparison of best versus worst clinical outcomes for adult cervical deformity surgery. Global Spine Journal. 2019;**9**(3):303-314

[6] Tang JA, Scheer JK, Smith JS, et al. The impact of standing regional cervical sagittal alignment on outcomes in posterior cervical fusion surgery. Neurosurgery. 2012;**71**(3):662-669; discussion 669

[7] Sullivan PW, Ghushchyan V. Preference-based EQ-5D index scores for chronic conditions in the United States. Medical Decision Making. 2006;**26**(4):410-420

[8] Vonck CE, Tanenbaum JE, Smith GA, et al. National Trends in demographics and outcomes following cervical fusion for cervical spondylotic myelopathy. Global Spine Journal. 2018;**8**(3):244-253

[9] Passias PG, Alas H, Lafage R, et al. Global spinal deformity from the upper cervical perspective. What is "abnormal" in the upper cervical spine? Journal of Craniovertebral Junction and Spine. 2019;**10**(3):152-159

[10] Kim HJ, Virk S, Elysee J, et al. The morphology of cervical deformities: A two-step cluster analysis to identify cervical deformity patterns. Journal of Neurosurgery. 2019;**15**:1-7

[11] Passias PG, Jalai CM, Worley N, et al. Development of new-onset cervical deformity in nonoperative adult spinal deformity patients with 2-year follow-up. International Journal of Spine Surgery. 2018;**12**(6):725-734

[12] Passias PG, Jalai CM, Lafage V, et al. Primary drivers of adult cervical deformity: Prevalence, variations in presentation, and effect of surgical treatment strategies on early postoperative alignment. Neurosurgery. 2018;**83**(4):651-659

[13] Protopsaltis TS, Lafage R, Vira S, et al. Novel angular measures of cervical deformity account for upper cervical compensation and sagittal alignment. Clinical Spine Surgery. 2017;**30**(7):E959-E967

[14] Ames CP, Smith JS, Eastlack R, et al. Reliability assessment of a novel cervical spine deformity classification system. Journal of Neurosurgery. 2015;**23**(6):673-683

[15] Scheer JK, Tang JA, Smith JS, et al. Cervical spine alignment, sagittal deformity, and clinical implications: A review. Journal of Neurosurgery. 2013;**19**(2):141-159

[16] Scheer JK, Ames CP, Deviren V. Assessment and treatment of cervical deformity. Neurosurgery Clinics of North America. 2013;**24**(2):249-274

[17] Ames CP, Smith JS, Scheer JK, et al. A standardized nomenclature for cervical spine soft-tissue release and osteotomy for deformity correction: Clinical article. Journal of Neurosurgery. 2013;**19**(3):269-278

[18] Tan LA, Riew KD, Traynelis VC. Cervical spine deformity-part 1: Biomechanics, radiographic parameters, and classification. Neurosurgery. 2017;**81**(2):197-203

[19] Beier G, Schuck M, Schuller E, et al. Determination of Physical Data of the Head I. Vol. 1979. Munich, West Germany: Center of Gravity and Moments of Inertia of Human Heads: Office of Naval Research; 1979. p. A333080

[20] Swartz EE, Floyd RT, Cendoma M. Cervical spine functional anatomy and the biomechanics of injury due to compressive loading. Journal of Athletic Training. 2005;**40**(3):155-161

[21] Bogduk N, Mercer S. Biomechanics of the cervical spine. I: Normal kinematics. Clinical Biomechanics (Bristol, Avon). 2000;**15**(9):633-648

[22] Panjabi M, Dvorak J, Duranceau J, et al. Three-dimensional movements of the upper cervical spine. Spine. 1988;**13**(7):726-730

[23] Pal GP, Sherk HH. The vertical stability of the cervical spine. Spine. 1988;**13**(5):447-449

[24] Lorenz M, Patwardhan A, Vanderby R Jr. Load-bearing characteristics of lumbar facets in normal and surgically altered spinal segments. Spine. 1983;**8**(2):122-130

[25] Nachemson A. Lumbar intradiscal pressure. Experimental studies on post-mortem material. Acta Orthopaedica Scandinavica. Supplementum. 1960;**43**:1-104

[26] Gay RE. The curve of the cervical spine: Variations and significance. Journal of Manipulative and Physiological Therapeutics. 1993;**16**(9):591-594

[27] McAviney J, Schulz D, Bock R, et al. Determining the relationship between cervical lordosis and neck complaints. Journal of Manipulative and Physiological Therapeutics. 2005;**28**(3):187-193

[28] Hardacker JW, Shuford RF, Capicotto PN, et al. Radiographic standing cervical segmental alignment in adult volunteers without neck symptoms. Spine. 1997;**22**(13):1472-1480; discussion 1480

[29] Gore DR. Roentgenographic findings in the cervical spine in asymptomatic persons: A ten-year follow-up. Spine. 2001;**26**(22):2463-2466

[30] Boyle JJ, Milne N, Singer KP. Influence of age on cervicothoracic spinal curvature: An *ex vivo* radiographic survey. Clinical Biomechanics (Bristol, Avon). 2002;**17**(5):361-367

[31] Gore DR, Sepic SB, Gardner GM. Roentgenographic findings of the cervical spine in asymptomatic people. Spine. 1986;**11**(6):521-524

[32] Takeshima T, Omokawa S, Takaoka T, et al. Sagittal alignment of

cervical flexion and extension: Lateral radiographic analysis. Spine. 2002;**27**(15):E348-E355

[33] Harrison DE, Harrison DD, Cailliet R, et al. Cobb method or Harrison posterior tangent method: Which to choose for lateral cervical radiographic analysis. Spine. 2000;**25**(16):2072-2078

[34] Jackson R. The Cervical Syndrome. 2d ed. Springfield, IL: Thomas; 1958

[35] Harrison DD. Chiropractic: The Physics of Spinal Correction: CBP Technique. Rev. ed. Harvest, Ala.? D.D. Harrison; 1994

[36] El Fegoun AB, Schwab F, Gamez L, et al. Center of gravity and radiographic posture analysis: A preliminary review of adult volunteers and adult patients affected by scoliosis. Spine. 2005;**30**(13):1535-1540

[37] Gangnet N, Pomero V, Dumas R, et al. Variability of the spine and pelvis location with respect to the gravity line: A three-dimensional stereoradiographic study using a force platform. Surgical and Radiologic Anatomy. 2003;**25**(5-6):424-433

[38] Lafage V, Schwab F, Skalli W, et al. Standing balance and sagittal plane spinal deformity: Analysis of spinopelvic and gravity line parameters. Spine. 2008;**33**(14):1572-1578

[39] Legaye J, Duval-Beaupere G. Gravitational forces and sagittal shape of the spine. Clinical estimation of their relations. International Orthopaedics. 2008;**32**(6):809-816

[40] Mac-Thiong JM, Transfeldt EE, Mehbod AA, et al. Can c7 plumbline and gravity line predict health related quality of life in adult scoliosis? Spine. 2009;**34**(15):E519-E527

[41] Schwab F, Lafage V, Boyce R, et al. Gravity line analysis in adult volunteers: Age-related correlation with spinal parameters, pelvic parameters, and foot position. Spine. 2006;**31**(25):E959-E967

[42] Zheng X, Chaudhari R, Wu C, et al. Repeatability test of C7 plumb line and gravity line on asymptomatic volunteers using an optical measurement technique. Spine. 2010;**35**(18):E889-E894

[43] Suk KS, Kim KT, Lee SH, et al. Significance of chin-brow vertical angle in correction of kyphotic deformity of ankylosing spondylitis patients. Spine. 2003;**28**(17):2001-2005

[44] Deviren V, Scheer JK, Ames CP. Technique of cervicothoracic junction pedicle subtraction osteotomy for cervical sagittal imbalance: Report of 11 cases. Journal of Neurosurgery. 2011;**15**(2):174-181

[45] Kim KT, Suk KS, Cho YJ, et al. Clinical outcome results of pedicle subtraction osteotomy in ankylosing spondylitis with kyphotic deformity. Spine. 2002;**27**(6):612-618

[46] Pigge RR, Scheerder FJ, Smit TH, et al. Effectiveness of preoperative planning in the restoration of balance and view in ankylosing spondylitis. Neurosurgical Focus. 2008;**24**(1):E7

[47] Wang Y, Zhang Y, Mao K, et al. Transpedicular bivertebrae wedge osteotomy and discectomy in lumbar spine for severe ankylosing spondylitis. Journal of Spinal Disorders & Techniques. 2010;**23**(3):186-191

[48] Kim KT, Lee SH, Son ES, et al. Surgical treatment of "chin-on-pubis" deformity in a patient with ankylosing spondylitis: A case report

of consecutive cervical, thoracic, and lumbar corrective osteotomies. Spine. 2012;**37**(16):E1017-E1021

[49] Schwab F, Ungar B, Blondel B, et al. Scoliosis Research Society-Schwab adult spinal deformity classification: A validation study. Spine. 2012;**37**(12):1077-1082

[50] Schwab FJ, Blondel B, Bess S, et al. Radiographical spinopelvic parameters and disability in the setting of adult spinal deformity: A prospective multicenter analysis. Spine. 2013;**38**(13):E803-E812

[51] Smith JS, Singh M, Klineberg E, et al. Surgical treatment of pathological loss of lumbar lordosis (flatback) in patients with normal sagittal vertical axis achieves similar clinical improvement as surgical treatment of elevated sagittal vertical axis. Journal of Neurosurgery. Spine. 2014;**21**(2):160-170

[52] Smith JS, Shaffrey CI, Fu KM, et al. Clinical and radiographic evaluation of the adult spinal deformity patient. Neurosurgery Clinics of North America. 2013;**24**(2):143-156

[53] Lee SH, Kim KT, Seo EM, et al. The influence of thoracic inlet alignment on the craniocervical sagittal balance in asymptomatic adults. Journal of Spinal Disorders & Techniques. 2012;**25**(2):E41-E47

[54] Tang JA, Scheer JK, Smith JS, Deviren V, Bess S, Hart RA, et al. The impact of standing regional cervical sagittal alignment on outcomes in posterior cervical fusion surgery. Neurosurgery. Sep 2012;**71**(3):662-669, discussion 669. DOI: 10.1227/NEU.0b013e31826100c9. PMID: 22653395

[55] Lee SH, Kim KT, Seo EM, Suk KS, Kwack YH, Son ES. The influence of thoracic inlet alignment on the craniocervical sagittal balance in asymptomatic adults. Journal of Spinal Disorders and Techniques. Apr 2012;**25**(2):E41-E47. DOI: 10.1097/BSD.0b013e3182396301. PMID: 22037167

[56] Blondel B, Schwab F, Ames CP, et al. The crucial role of cervical alignment in regulating sagittal spino-pelvic alignment in human standing posture. In: The 19th International Meeting on Advanced Spine Techniques, Istanbul, Turkey. Denver, CO: International Spine Study Group; 2012

[57] Jackson RP, McManus AC. Radiographic analysis of sagittal plane alignment and balance in standing volunteers and patients with low back pain matched for age, sex, and size. A prospective controlled clinical study. Spine. 1994;**19**(14):1611-1618

[58] Bernhardt M, Bridwell KH. Segmental analysis of the sagittal plane alignment of the normal thoracic and lumbar spines and thoracolumbar junction. Spine. 1989;**14**(7):717-721

[59] Wang VY, Chou D. The cervicothoracic junction. Neurosurgery Clinics of North America. 2007;**18**(2):365-371

[60] An HS, Vaccaro A, Cotler JM, et al. Spinal disorders at the cervicothoracic junction. Spine. 1994;**19**(22):2557-2564

[61] Knott PT, Mardjetko SM, Techy F. The use of the T1 sagittal angle in predicting overall sagittal balance of the spine. The Spine Journal. 2010;**10**(11):994-998

[62] Steinmetz MP, Stewart TJ, Kager CD, et al. Cervical deformity correction. Neurosurgery. 2007;**60**(Suppl. 1): S90-S97

[63] Iyer S, Lenke LG, Nemani VM, et al. Variations in occipitocervical and cervicothoracic alignment parameters based on age: A prospective study of asymptomatic volunteers using full-body radiographs. Spine. 2016;**41**(23):1837-1844

[64] Song K, Su X, Zhang Y, et al. Optimal chin-brow vertical angle for sagittal visual fields in ankylosing spondylitis kyphosis. European Spine Journal. 2016;**25**(8):2596-2604

[65] Tan LA, Riew KD, Traynelis VC. Cervical spine deformity-part 2: Management algorithm and anterior techniques. Neurosurgery. 2017;**81**(4):561-567

[66] Umapathi T, Chaudhry V, Cornblath D, et al. Head drop and camptocormia. Journal of Neurology, Neurosurgery, and Psychiatry. 2002;**73**(1):1-7

[67] Ames CP, Blondel B, Scheer JK, et al. Cervical radiographical alignment: Comprehensive assessment techniques and potential importance in cervical myelopathy. Spine. 2013;**38**(22 Suppl. 1): S149-S160

[68] Albert TJ, Vacarro A. Postlaminectomy kyphosis. Spine. 1998;**23**(24):2738-2745

[69] Deutsch H, Haid RW, Rodts GE, et al. Postlaminectomy cervical deformity. Neurosurgical Focus. 2003;**15**(3):E5

[70] Jarzem PF, Quance DR, Doyle DJ, et al. Spinal cord tissue pressure during spinal cord distraction in dogs. Spine. 1992;**17**(Suppl. 8):S227-S234

[71] Tachibana S, Kitahara Y, Iida H, et al. Spinal cord intramedullary pressure. A possible factor in syrinx growth. Spine. 1994;**19**(19):2174-2178; discussion 2178-2179

[72] Iida H, Tachibana S. Spinal cord intramedullary pressure: Direct cord traction test. Neurologia Medico-Chirurgica (Tokyo). 1995;**35**(2):75-77

[73] Kitahara Y, Iida H, Tachibana S. Effect of spinal cord stretching due to head flexion on intramedullary pressure. Neurologia Medico-Chirurgica (Tokyo). 1995;**35**(5):285-288

[74] Shimizu K, Nakamura M, Nishikawa Y, et al. Spinal kyphosis causes demyelination and neuronal loss in the spinal cord: A new model of kyphotic deformity using juvenile Japanese small game fowls. Spine. 2005;**30**(21):2388-2392

[75] Smith JS, Lafage V, Ryan DJ, et al. Association of myelopathy scores with cervical sagittal balance and normalized spinal cord volume: Analysis of 56 preoperative cases from the AOSpine North America myelopathy study. Spine. 2013;**38**(22 Suppl. 1):S161-S170

[76] Wade R, Yang H, McKenna C, et al. A systematic review of the clinical effectiveness of EOS 2D/3D X-ray imaging system. European Spine Journal. 2013;**22**(2):296-304

[77] Wybier M, Bossard P. Musculoskeletal imaging in progress: The EOS imaging system. Joint, bone, spine. revue Du Rhumatisme. 2013;**80**(3):238-243

[78] Al-Aubaidi Z, Lebel D, Oudjhane K, et al. Three-dimensional imaging of the spine using the EOS system: Is it reliable? A comparative study using computed tomography imaging. Journal of Pediatric Orthopedics. Part B. 2013;**22**(5):409-412

[79] Somoskeoy S, Tunyogi-Csapo M, Bogyo C, et al. Accuracy and reliability of coronal and sagittal spinal curvature data based on patient-specific

three-dimensional models created by the EOS 2D/3D imaging system. The Spine Journal. 2012;**12**(11):1052-1059

[80] Lazennec JY, Brusson A, Rousseau MA. Hip-spine relations and sagittal balance clinical consequences. European Spine Journal. 2011;**20**(Suppl. 5):686-698

[81] Obeid I, Hauger O, Aunoble S, et al. Global analysis of sagittal spinal alignment in major deformities: Correlation between lack of lumbar lordosis and flexion of the knee. European Spine Journal. 2011;**20**(Suppl. 5):681-685

[82] Etame AB, Than KD, Wang AC, et al. Surgical management of symptomatic cervical or cervicothoracic kyphosis due to ankylosing spondylitis. Spine. 2008;**33**(16):E559-E564

[83] Smith JS, Shaffrey CI, Lafage V, et al. Spontaneous improvement of cervical alignment after correction of global sagittal balance following pedicle subtraction osteotomy. Journal of Neurosurgery. 2012;**17**(4):300-307

[84] Ha Y, Schwab F, Lafage V, et al. Reciprocal changes in cervical spine alignment after corrective thoracolumbar deformity surgery. European Spine Journal. 2014;**23**(3):552-559

[85] Smith JS, Lafage V, Schwab FJ, et al. Prevalence and type of cervical deformity among 470 adults with throacolumbar deformity. Spine (Phila Pa 1976). 2014;**39**(17):E1001-E1009

[86] Smith JS, Klineberg E, Schwab F, et al. Change in classification grade by the SRS-Schwab adult spinal deformity classification predicts impact on health-related quality of life measures: Prospective analysis of operative and nonoperative treatment. Spine. 2013;**38**(19):1663-1671

[87] Terran J, Schwab F, Shaffrey CI, et al. The SRS-Schwab adult spinal deformity classification: Assessment and clinical correlations based on a prospective operative and nonoperative cohort. Neurosurgery. 2013;**73**(4):559-568

[88] Acosta FL Jr, Aryan HE, Ames CP. Successful outcome of six-level cervicothoracic corpectomy and circumferential reconstruction: Case report and review of literature on multilevel cervicothoracic corpectomy. European Spine Journal. 2006;**15**(Suppl. 5):670-674

[89] Acosta FL Jr, Aryan HE, Chou D, et al. Long-term biomechanical stability and clinical improvement after extended multilevel corpectomy and circumferential reconstruction of the cervical spine using titanium mesh cages. Journal of Spinal Disorders & Techniques. 2008;**21**(3):165-174

[90] Aryan HE, Sanchez-Mejia RO, Ben-Haim S, et al. Successful treatment of cervical myelopathy with minimal morbidity by circumferential decompression and fusion. European Spine Journal. 2007;**16**(9):1401-1409

[91] Guinn JMV, Pennicooke B, Rivera J, Mummaneni PV, Chou D. Anterior cervical discectomy with fusion and plating for correction of degenerative cervical kyphosis: 2-dimensional operative video. Operative Neurosurgery Hagerstown Md. 2021;**20**(3):E214. DOI: 10.1093/ons/opaa339

[92] Gillis CC, Kaszuba MC, Traynelis VC. Cervical radiographic parameters in 1- and 2-level anterior cervical discectomy and fusion. Journal of Neurosurgery. Spine. 2016;**25**(4):421-429. DOI: 10.3171/2016.2.SPINE151056

[93] Smith GW, Robinson RA. The treatment of certain cervical-spine

disorders by anterior removal of the intervertebral disc and interbody fusion. The Journal of Bone and Joint Surgery. American Volume. 1958;**40-A**(3):607-624

[94] Sasso RC, Ruggiero RA, Reilly TM, Hall PV. Early reconstruction failures after multilevel cervical corpectomy. Spine. 2003;**28**(2):140-142. DOI: 10.1097/00007632-200301150-00009

[95] Vaccaro AR, Falatyn SP, Scuderi GJ, et al. Early failure of long segment anterior cervical plate fixation. Journal of Spinal Disorders. 1998;**11**(5):410-415

[96] Safaee MM, Tan LA, Riew KD. Anterior osteotomy for rigid cervical deformity correction. Journal of Spine Surgery Hong Kong. 2020;**6**(1):210-216. DOI: 10.21037/jss.2019.12.10

[97] Kim HJ, Piyaskulkaew C, Riew KD. Anterior cervical osteotomy for fixed cervical deformities. Spine. 2014;**39**(21):1751-1757. DOI: 10.1097/BRS.0000000000000502

[98] Simmons ED, DiStefano RJ, Zheng Y, Simmons EH. Thirty-six years experience of cervical extension osteotomy in ankylosing spondylitis: Techniques and outcomes. Spine (Phila Pa 1976). 2006;**31**(26):3006-3012. DOI: 10.1097/01.brs.0000250663.12224.d9

[99] Langeloo DD, Journee HL, Pavlov PW, de Kleuver M. Cervical osteotomy in ankylosing spondylitis: Evaluation of new developments. European Spine Journal. 2006;**15**(4):493-500. DOI: 10.1007/s00586-005-0945-z

[100] Tokala DP, Lam KS, Freeman BJC, Webb JK. C7 decancellisation closing wedge osteotomy for the correction of fixed cervico-thoracic kyphosis. European Spine Journal. 2007;**16**(9):1471-1478. DOI: 10.1007/s00586-006-0290-x

[101] Mummaneni PV, Dhall SS, Rodts GE, Haid RW. Circumferential fusion for cervical kyphotic deformity. Journal of Neurosurgery. Spine. 2008;**9**(6):515-521. DOI: 10.3171/SPI.2008.10.08226

[102] Etame AB, Wang AC, Than KD, La Marca F, Park P. Outcomes after surgery for cervical spine deformity: Review of the literature. Neurosurgical Focus. 2010;**28**(3):E14. DOI: 10.3171/2010.1.FOCUS09278

[103] Belanger TA, Milam RA, Roh JS, Bohlman HH. Cervicothoracic extension osteotomy for chin-on-chest deformity in ankylosing spondylitis. The Journal of Bone and Joint Surgery. American Volume. 2005;**87**(8):1732-1738. DOI: 10.2106/JBJS.C.01472

[104] Kim CW, Hyun SJ, Kim KJ. Surgical impact on global sagittal alignment and health-related quality of life following cervical kyphosis correction surgery: Systematic review. Neurospine. 2020;**17**(3):497-504. DOI: 10.14245/ns.2040476.238

[105] Passias PG, Horn SR, Jalai CM, et al. Comparative analysis of perioperative complications between a multicenter prospective cervical deformity database and the Nationwide inpatient sample database. The Spine Journal. 2017;**17**(11):1633-1640

[106] Smith JS, Ramchandran S, Lafage V, et al. Prospective multicenter assessment of early complication rates associated with adult cervical deformity surgery in 78 patients. Neurosurgery. 2016;**79**(3):378-388

[107] Smith JS, Shaffrey CI, Lafage R, et al. Three-column osteotomy for correction of cervical and cervicothoracic deformities: Alignment changes and early complications in

a multicenter prospective series of 23 patients. European Spine Journal. 2017;**26**(8):2128-2137

[108] Lafage R, Smith JS, Soroceanu A, et al. Predicting mechanical failure following cervical deformity surgery: A composite score integrating age-adjusted cervical alignment targets. Global Spine Journal. 2022;**13**:2432-2438

[109] Passias PG, Horn SR, Oh C, et al. Predicting the occurrence of postoperative distal junctional kyphosis in cervical deformity patients. Neurosurgery. 2020;**86**(1):E38-E46

[110] Safaee MM, Deviren V, Dalle Ore C, et al. Ligament augmentation for prevention of proximal junctional kyphosis and proximal junctional failure in adult spinal deformity. Journal of Neurosurgery. 2018;**28**(5):512-519

[111] Passias PG, Alas H, Pierce KE, et al. The impact of the lower instrumented level on outcomes in cervical deformity surgery. Journal of Craniovertebral Junction and Spine. 2021;**12**(3):306-310

Chapter 6

Spinal Deformities in Spinal Dysraphia Syndrome

Sergey O. Ryabykh, Olga M. Sergeenko, Alexander V. Gubin, Ilkhom E. Khujanazarov, Vladimir S. Klimov, Dmitry Y. Zinenko, Alexey A. Kalashnikov, Evgenia M. Berdichevskaya and Timur A. Dzhumatov

Abstract

Progressive spinal deformity is a significant comorbidity associated with MMC. It leads to loss of truncal height and causes sitting, breathing, eating, and urination difficulties due to increased chest and abdominal pressures. Spinal deformities associated with MMC can be divided into 2 major groups: predominantly neuromuscular kyphoscoliosis or lordoscoliosis and severe rigid kyphosis or sharp-angled kyphosis. Kyphoscoliosis is a common finding in patients with thoracolumbar myelodysplasia, whereas lordoscoliosis is more common in patients with cauda equina and conus medullaris dysplasia. Early surgical correction improves body balance and quality of life and helps reduce the aggressiveness of surgical intervention. The dual growing rod technique is safe and effective in cases of moderate neuromuscular kyphoscoliosis or lordoscoliosis at an early age. Kyphectomy is a challenging procedure with high rates of complications, especially skin problems, but in patients with significant rigid kyphosis, there are no viable alternative procedures.

Keywords: myelomeningocele, myeloschisis, neural tube defects, MMC-related kyphosis, post MMC syndrome, caudal regression, myelocele, post MMS-related kyphosis, caudal regression syndrome

1. Introduction

Spinal deformities are frequently observed in myelomeningocele (MMC) patients. Scoliosis, for instance, manifests in approximately 94% of thoracolumbar MMC cases and encompasses around 52% of cases overall. The prevalence of kyphosis stands at 10–20%, while lumbar hyperlordosis occurs in 1.5% of cases.

Progressive spinal deformity stands out as a significant comorbidity associated with MMC. It leads to a reduction in trunk height, giving rise to challenges in sitting, breathing, eating, and urination due to heightened chest and abdominal pressures. These deformities are rooted in neuromuscular disruptions and vertebral anomalies. Spinal deformities linked with MMC can be classified into two major categories: primarily neuromuscular kyphoscoliosis or lordoscoliosis, and severe rigid kyphosis

IntechOpen

or sharply angled kyphosis. Kyphoscoliosis commonly presents in patients with thoracolumbar myelodysplasia, whereas lordoscoliosis is more prevalent among those with cauda equina and conus medullaris dysplasia.

Bracing for patients with MMC and spinal deformities often proves ineffective, potentially leading to rib deformation, diminished respiratory capacity, and neuropathic skin ulcers. In contrast, early surgical correction holds the promise of enhancing body balance, quality of life, and reducing the need for more aggressive surgical interventions.

The dual growing rod technique emerges as both safe and effective for cases involving moderate neuromuscular kyphoscoliosis or lordoscoliosis at an early age, although it is accompanied by a notable incidence of rod fractures. On the other hand, kyphectomy presents as a demanding procedure with elevated complication rates, particularly skin-related issues. However, for patients grappling with significant rigid kyphosis, viable alternative procedures remain scarce.

In the following account, we share our experiences working with patients harboring diverse types of MMC-related spinal deformities. This account centers on the prompt correction of deformities via the dual growing rod technique and instrumented fusion, sometimes involving vertebrectomy. Notably, only a handful of studies have outlined successful treatments for MMC-related spinal deformities and their long-term outcomes.

2. General information

The term "spinal dysraphia" or "spinal dysraphia syndrome" and its accompanying anatomical characteristics were initially introduced by the German pathologist F.D. von Recklinghausen in 1886. This groundbreaking terminology comprehensively encompassed all variations of both closed and open neural tube defects (NTDs). Fast-forward to the year 2000, when P. Tortori-Donati et al. further elucidated and systematically categorized the primary forms of spinal dysgraphia [1]. Newer classifications of NTDs refer to the basics of embryonic development in an attempt to separate these abnormalities depending on the stage of their occurrence (gastrulation, primary neurulation, junctional neurulation, and secondary neurulation) [2].

NTDs occur on average in 1 out of every 1000 newborns [3]. Among these cases, open forms are observed in an average of 4.7 out of every 100,000 newborns [4, 5].

Myelomeningocele (MMC), also referred to as an open neural tube defect (NTD), stands as the most prevalent form of neural tube abnormalities. An additional variant within the realm of open NTDs is myeloschisis. Myeloschisis, alongside the classical thoracolumbar and lumbar MMCs, arises during the primary neurulation phase due to disrupted apposition, fusion, and neuroectodermal disjunction that transpires in the third to fourth week of embryonic development. A segment of MMC cases, specifically those presenting as sacral forms below the S1 level, has recently been associated with disorders of secondary neurulation. This attribution stems from distinct clinical symptoms observed in these patients, setting them apart from the primary group [5]. MMC and myeloschisis represent the predominant presentation within the spectrum of NTDs, accounting for approximately 80% of all cases. Estimates place the prevalence of this type of NTDs between 3.4 and 4.6 cases per 10,000 live births, underscoring its significance in the realm of congenital anomalies [4, 6].

Eubanks J.D. and Cheruvu V.K. discuss the prevalence, which stands at 12% of the population. The majority of these cases manifest as asymptomatic forms, often detected incidentally during MRI and CT scans in patients [3]. The group of so-called closed NTSs is diverse and extensive, encompassing presumed gastulation defects (such as split cord malformations and neuroenteric cysts and tracts), primary neurulation defects (type 1 spinal lipomas, limited dorsal myeloschisis), junctional neurulation defects (junctional neural tube defect, type 2 spinal lipomas, and segmental spinal dysgeneses), and early and late secondary neurulation defects (type 3 and 4 lipomas, retained conus medullaris, sacral meningocele, dermal sinuses) [7]. While this embryonic classification certainly sparks debates and discussions, it presents a logical structure and holds practical utility.

All spinal deformities in patients with NTDs contribute to issues concerning respiration, digestion, and urination due to heightened intra-abdominal pressure and elevated position of the diaphragmatic dome.

One facet of comprehensive rehabilitation for patients affected by severe forms of spinal dysraphia involves managing and treating the manifestations of post-MMC syndrome. This syndrome embodies an array of pathological effects stemming from spinal lesions, materializing as deformities of varying forms, intensities, and intricate courses. As a result, patients exhibit distinct prognoses, necessitate tailored social support, and call for personalized surgical interventions. Our endeavor has been to outline the fundamental principles for managing such treatments.

3. General terminology

See **Table 1**.

Vertebral syndrome	A compilation of clinical and radiological symptoms that define the anatomical condition (structure, shape) and functional alterations in the spine, spinal canal, and spinal cord
Vertebrogenic syndrome	A compilation of intricate clinical and neurological (motor, sensory, visceral, autonomic), positional (postural), and radiological symptoms, originating from pathogenetic alterations in the anatomy and functionality of the spine and spinal cord
Consequences of MMC and mieloshysis (post-myelomeningocele syndrome, post-MMC syndrome)	A compilation of comprehensive clinical (orthopedic, neurological, adaptive) and radiological symptoms that depict the aftermath of surgical interventions for diverse forms of ONTDs
Dysraphic syndrome (Synonym: Bremer syndrome, spinal dysraphia syndrome, dysraphic complex (status), dysraphic myelodysplasia, dysraphia, Fuchs myelodysraphia)	The overarching term for developmental anomalies distinguished by the absence of fusion among anatomical structures along the body's midline
Spinal dysraphia (vertebral component of Bremer's syndrome)	A term employed to describe the incomplete fusion or absence of fusion of midline structures, including vertebrae, spinal canal, and spinal cord

Table 1.
Basic syndromic terminology [1, 8, 9].

4. Nosological groups according to ICD-11

LA02 Spina bifida.
LA02.0 Spina bifida cystica.
LA02.00 Myelomeningocele with hydrocephalus.
LA02.01 Myelomeningocele without hydrocephalus.
LA02.02 Myelocystocele.
LA02.0Y Other specified spina bifida cystica.
LA02.0Z Spina bifida cystica, unspecified.
LA02.1 Spina bifida aperta.
LA02.Y Other specified spina bifida.
LA02.Z Spina bifida, unspecified.
LA07 Structural developmental anomalies of the neurenteric canal, spinal cord or vertebral column.
LA07.0 Primary tethered cord syndrome.
LA07.1 Diastematomyelia.
LA07.2 Amyelia.
LA07.3 Primary syringomyelia or hydromyelia.
LA07.4 Arnold-Chiari malformation type I.

Orthopedic	• Spinal deformities • Deformities of the lower extremities • Dislocations and contractures of lower extremity joints, particularly the hip • Clubfoot, including cases recurring after treatment • Osteoporosis • Fractures of long bones in the lower extremities, including instances of recurrence
Neurological and neurosurgical	• Paresis and paralysis • Tethered spinal cord syndrome • Hydrosyringomyelia • Arnold-Chiari malformation
X-ray	• Posterior column maldevelopment, ranging from partial to complete absence of vertebral arches • Vertebrae anomalies (including failure of formation, fusion, and segmentation) • Spinal deformities—encompassing kyphosis, scoliosis, kyphoscoliosis; as well as lordoscoliosis • Various forms of myelodysplasia, encompassing conditions both at the spina bifida level and within the craniovertebral junction region
Other clinical manifestations	• Skin indicators positioned along the spine—hypertrichosis, pigmented spots, retraction, and subcutaneous lipomas; • Pressure ulcers occurring at the peak of kyphotic deformity • Impaired functionality of pelvic organs • Persistent urinary tract infections • Respiratory insufficiency attributed to an elevated diaphragmatic dome and diminished chest volume

Table 2.
Clinical and radiation manifestations of spinal dysraphia syndrome [10–14].

LB73.0 Occult spinal dysraphism.
LA07.Y Other specified structural developmental anomalies of the neurenteric canal, spinal cord, or vertebral column.
LA07.Z Structural developmental anomalies of the neurenteric canal, spinal cord, or vertebral column, unspecified (**Table 2**).

5. Clinical and radiation features of vertebral syndrome in ONTDs

- Absence of posterior vertebral structures (spina bifida) [8, 11, 15–34]
- Broadened vertebral canal
- Flattening of vertebral bodies
- Reduced bone density
- Hypoplasia of the sacrum and pelvis or sacral agenesis
- Scar tissue changes at the apex of the deformity
- Soft tissue deficiency, leading to pressure ulcers at the apex of the deformity
- Predominance of combined kyphosis due to the interplay of congenital anomalies and neurogenic factors
- Pelvic rotation
- Tethered spinal cord and myelodysplasia (paresis)
- Resistance to conservative treatment methods

6. Spinal deformities in closed NTDs

The prevalence of congenital vertebral anomalies or scoliosis varies according to the type of closed NTD. For instance, in cases of split cord malformations (SCM), disturbances in spinal segmentation (like hemivertebra, butterfly vertebra, and

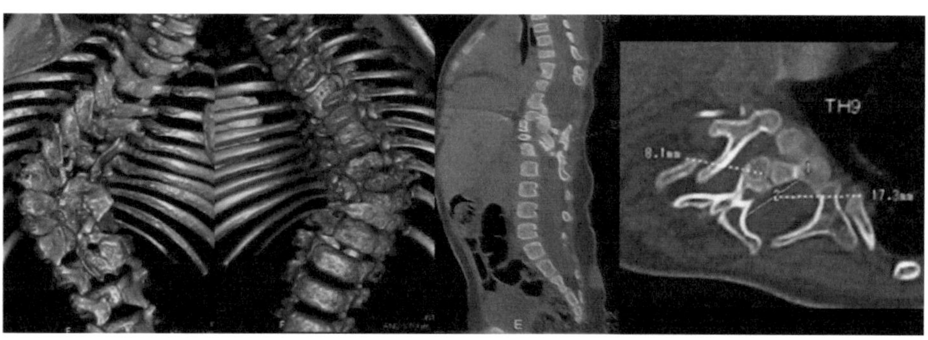

Figure 1.
CT scan of the thoracic and lumbar spine of a 17-month-old child with multiply segmentation disorders, split cord malformation type 1 at the level of Th11-L1.

unsegmented bar) are frequently encountered (**Figure 1**) [35, 36]. This occurrence may be attributed to the likelihood that these anomalies originate during the early phases of embryonic development.

Segmental spinal dysgenesis falls under disruptions of the junctional neurulation stage and is characterized by localized spinal cord thinning, with the underlying conus medullaris and segmental vertebral agenesis in the thoracolumbar transition area—typically without associated anomalies (**Figure 2**). In spinal cord lipomas, vertebral segmentation irregularities are rarely encountered, usually presenting with spina bifida only. Notably, the Currarino syndrome holds a distinct position, where

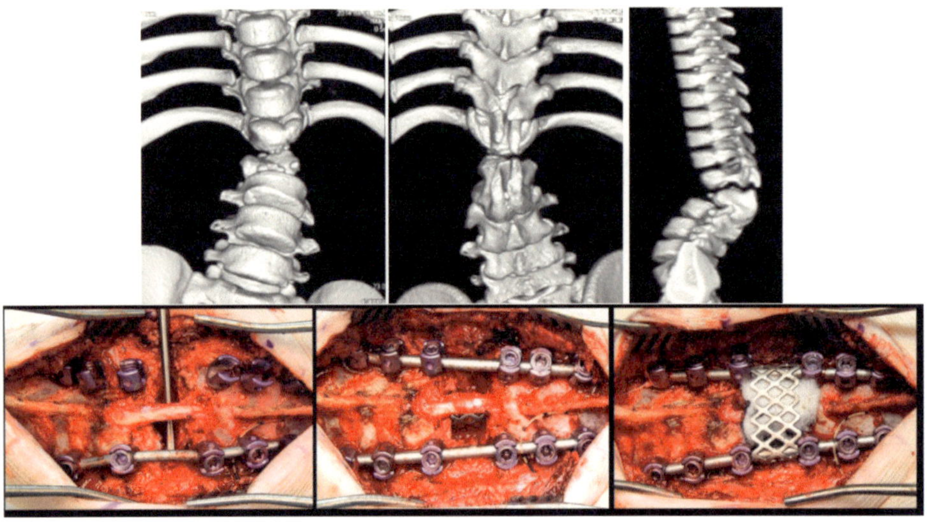

Figure 2.
CT scan and surgical treatment of the spine of a 6-year-old child with segmental spinal dysgenesis.

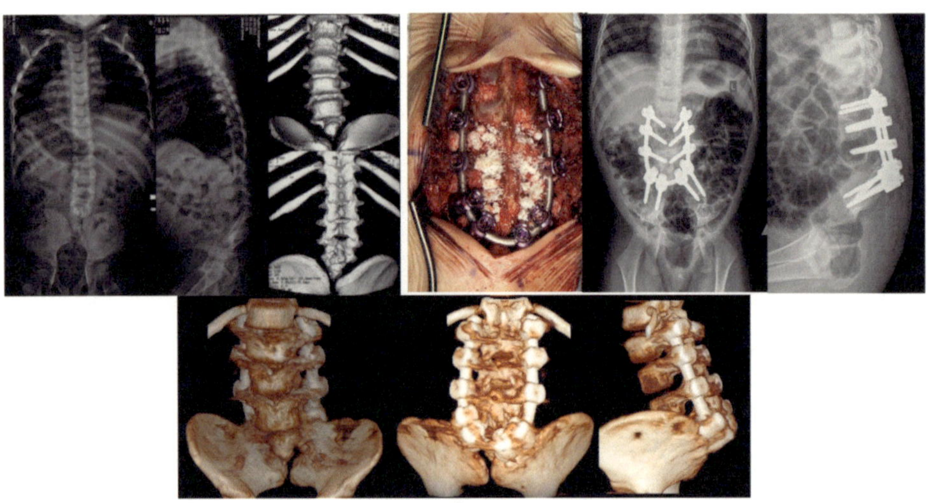

b

Figure 3.
Surgical management for lumbo-sacral agenesis.

developmental anomalies of the caudal spinal cord region (such as filum terminalis lipoma) coincide with agenesis of the lower sacrum (**Figure 3**).

7. Spinal deformities in open NTDS

Spinal deformities resulting in ONTDs are not uncommon; however, the degree of deformity aligns with both the extent of the dysraphic level and the concurrent spinal anomalies. In the cervical spine, open NTDs are situated in 2–5% of cases; within the thoracic region, the prevalence is around 2–3%; in the lumbar region, it accounts for 25%; and in the lumbosacral area, the majority, comprising 65–70%, of open NTDs

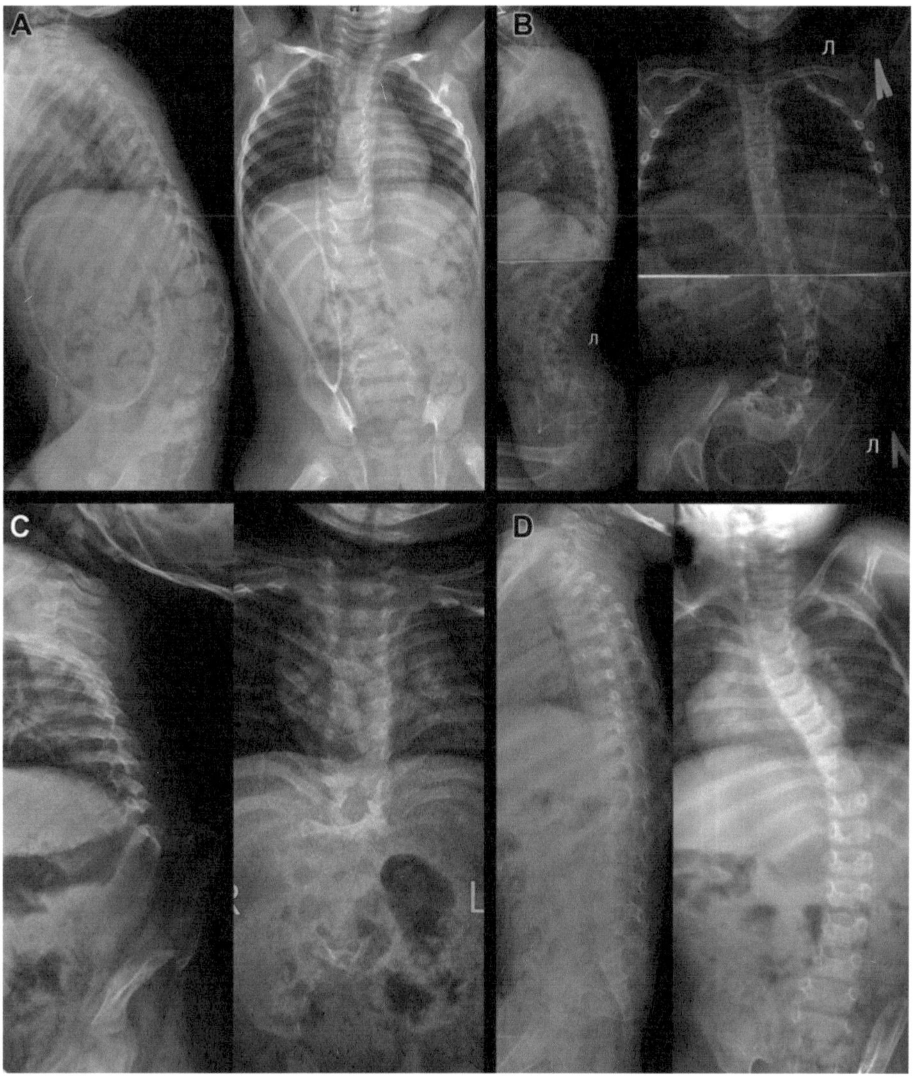

Figure 4.
Lateral and anteroposterior radiographs of four patients showcasing diverse types of spinal deformities associated with myelomeningocele: (A) kyphoscoliosis; (B) lordoscoliosis; (C) pronounced lumbar kyphosis; (D) scoliosis and "flatback" spine.

are localized [1, 4, 8, 9]. The neurological level of the lesion stands as a pivotal factor that impacts mobility, functional-motor capacity, the development of secondary orthopedic complications, their treatment, overall outcome, and eventual prognosis.

Spinal deformities are prevalent among individuals with open NTDs. Scoliosis and lordoscoliosis are observed in 52% of cases and in 94% of patients with thoracolumbar open NTDs. The occurrence of kyphosis stands at 20%, while lumbar hyperlordosis is encountered in 1.5% of cases [6, 11, 14, 21, 26, 37]. These deformities can be instigated by a denervation (paralytic) component, vertebral anomalies, or frequently, a combination of both [15, 21, 22, 29, 37–42]. Spinal deformities linked to open neural tube defects (NTDs) can be categorized into two major groups: predominantly neuromuscular kypho- or lordoscoliosis (**Figure 4a** and **b**), and distinct rigid kyphosis or acute-angled kyphosis (**Figure 4c**). The kyphoscoliotic variant of deformity is more prevalent among patients with thoracolumbar myelodysplasia, while lordoscoliosis is commonly observed in lower (lumbar and sacral) ONTDs.

Progression of the deformity is a characteristic feature of open NTDs, resulting in a decrease in body height, compromised upright posture, and challenges with respiration, digestion, and urination due to heightened intra-abdominal pressure and elevated position of the diaphragmatic dome [18].

Almost always, with kyphotic deformity, the vertebrae at the apex of the deformity are wedge-shaped, and in severe forms of acute-angled kyphosis with ulcer at the apex, there may be a complete absence of one or two vertebrae.

Neuromuscular deformities affecting the hips, ankles, and feet in patients with open NTDs commonly present as contractures, subluxations, or dislocations. These deformities can contribute to, or exacerbate, pelvic tilt and spinal misalignment. Furthermore, patients with open NTDs frequently experience torsional deformities in the lower extremities, impacting the femur and/or lower legs.

Objectives of surgical intervention for spinal deformities in open NTDs [42–44].

- Rectification of deformity and reestablishment of trunk equilibrium
- Restoration of upright stance capability
- Enhancement of lung capacity (SAL) and abdominal space
- Diminished stress on the spinal cord in fixed spinal cord syndrome (through kyphosis correction with shortening osteotomy)
- Amplification of manual dexterity
- Addressing and thwarting pressure ulcers at the apex
- Augmenting urinary passage by alleviating intra-abdominal pressure
- Advancing patient care
- Elevating the quality of life for patients and their caregivers
- Extending life expectancy

See **Table 3**.

Characteristics of spinal deformity	Features of orthopedic correction
Mobile scoliosis, lordoscoliosis, and kyphoscoliosis without asymmetrical vertebral segmentation disorders (**Figures 5** and **6**) [21]	Growth-friendly systems (dual growing rods, VEPTR) for Risser 0–3 [16, 21–24, 38] Deformity correction with Schwab I-II osteotomy for Risser 4 Closely monitor fixed spinal cord syndrome
Rigid deformities with congenital component—hemivertebra, asymmetrical butterfly vertebrae, asymmetrical unsegmented bar, acute-angle kyphosis, no depend on Risser (**Figure 7**) [21]	Vertebrectomy Schwab III-VI + short posterior spine fusion [15, 21–24, 30, 37] Indirect treatment of spinal cord fixation by shortening the length of the spinal column
Deformities complicated by infected bedsores (usually at the apex of kyphosis) (**Figure 8**) [21, 36, 45]	Two-stage surgical treatment: Stage 1—external temporary fixation (halo-pelvic, transpedicular-pelvic) for stage distraction; Stage 2—kyphectomy with posterior spine fusion [21, 36, 45].

Table 3.
Options for surgical correction of open NTDs-related deformities, taking into account the characteristics of the pathology of the spine.

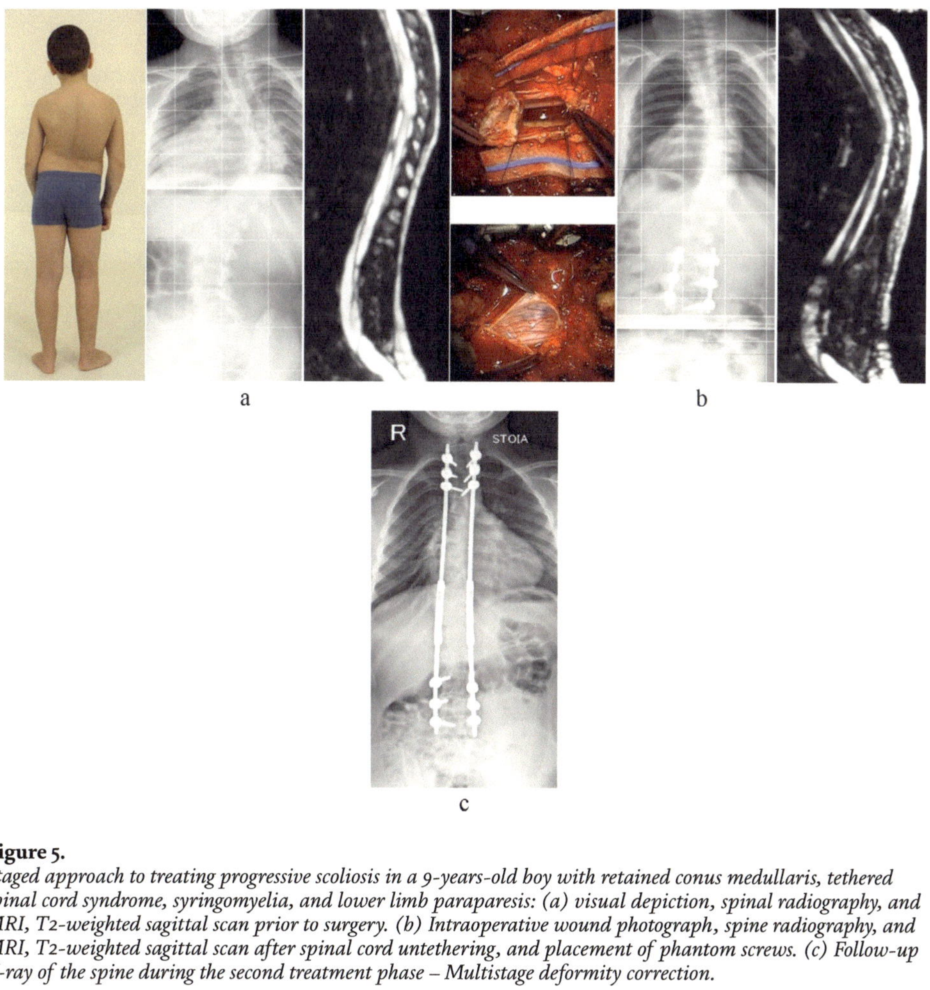

Figure 5.
Staged approach to treating progressive scoliosis in a 9-years-old boy with retained conus medullaris, tethered spinal cord syndrome, syringomyelia, and lower limb paraparesis: (a) visual depiction, spinal radiography, and MRI, T2-weighted sagittal scan prior to surgery. (b) Intraoperative wound photograph, spine radiography, and MRI, T2-weighted sagittal scan after spinal cord untethering, and placement of phantom screws. (c) Follow-up X-ray of the spine during the second treatment phase – Multistage deformity correction.

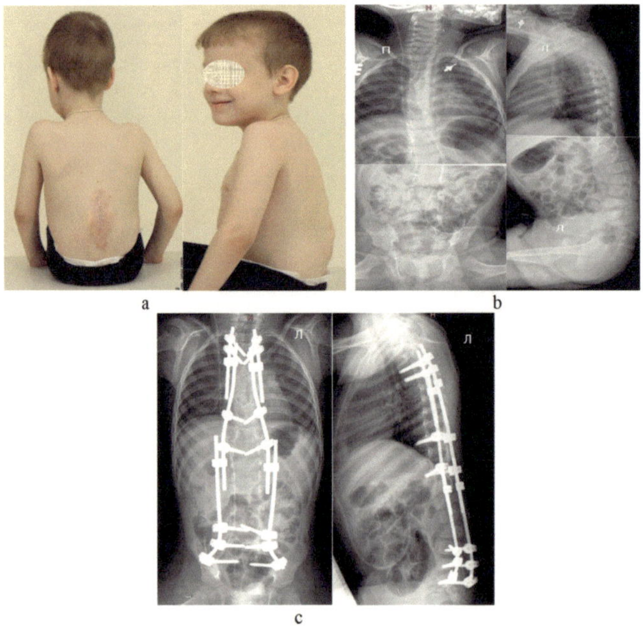

Figure 6.
Illustrations of treatment for mobile spinal deformities in patient with post-MMC deformity. (a) Depiction of a 5-year-old child's appearance; (b) spine X-ray before surgery; (c) spine X-ray after the implantation of dual growing rod system.

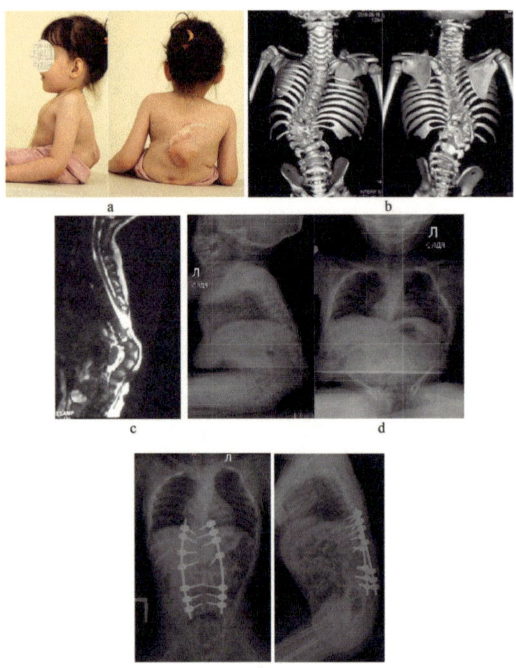

Figure 7.
Correction of a rigid spinal deformity in an 18-month-old child with post-myeloshysis severe kyphosis. (a) Child's preoperative appearance, (b) CT scan, and (c) MRI before surgery; (d) intraoperative photographs; (e) spinal X-ray after surgery.

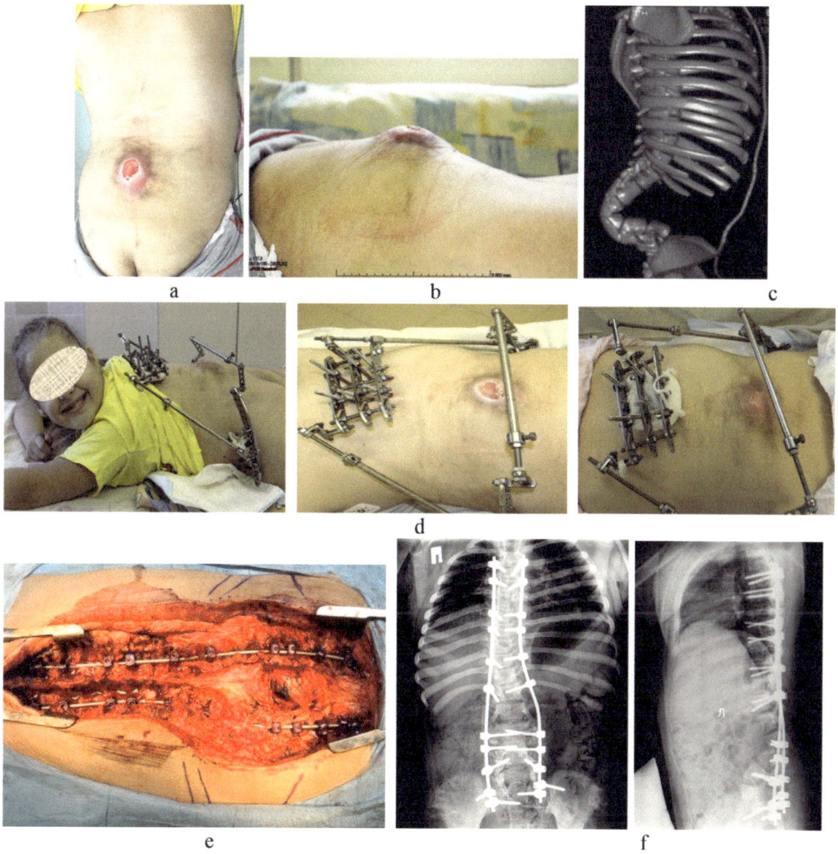

Figure 8.
Staged surgical treatment of post-myeloshysis spinal deformity complicated by recurrent bedsore in a 9-year-old child. Appearance of the child (a, b) and CT scan of the spine (d) before the surgical treatment; (c) appearance at the stages of treatment in the external fixation frame; (e) intraoperative photos; (f) X-rays of the spine after kyphectomy with posterior spinal-pelvic fixation.

Important Note: Employing spinal-pelvic fixation for correcting post-open NTDs deformities enhances spinal stability. Nevertheless, in younger children, it could potentially correlate with the incomplete maturation of supporting bone structures due to their diminutive size, spatial arrangement, and strength. Consequently, the decision to extend spinal-pelvic fixation may be deferred from the primary intervention to a subsequent phase during ongoing child monitoring (refer to the "Complications and Prevention" section for further details).

8. Constraints on the surgical correction of spinal deformities within the context of spinal dysraphia syndrome

The primary objectives of surgical rehabilitation for patients with spinal deformities stemming from spinal dysraphia syndrome encompass the enhancement of the child's quality of life, facilitation of social integration, and the enablement of proper care. Consequently, surgical intervention may be contraindicated under the following circumstances:

Complication	Frequency (%)	Prevention methods	Treatment
Wound failure	10	Precise closure of the wound involves delicately aligning the edges without imposing tension, and whenever feasible, considering scar excision	If conservative treatment is ineffective and there is a risk of construct exposure, soft tissue reconstruction involving a plastic surgeon is considered
Implant-related complications (more often—dislocation of hooks and screws)	15	Thorough preoperative strategizing. Thorough evaluation of the dimensions of the underlying bones relevant to their respective structural components. Comprehensive evaluation of the strength of supporting bones, with particular emphasis on the caudal elements such as the sacrum and pelvis. Strategizing for pivotal surgical interventions	Re-do surgery
Surgical site infection	5	Preoperative rehabilitation of foci of chronic infection (primarily urinary). Active drainage of the wound, evacuation of hematoma and serous contents. Adequate antibiotic therapy. Prevention of bedsores.	Early re-do surgery

Table 4.
*Complications of surgical treatment of spinal deformities in patients with open NTDs (**Figure 9**) [21, 46–50].*

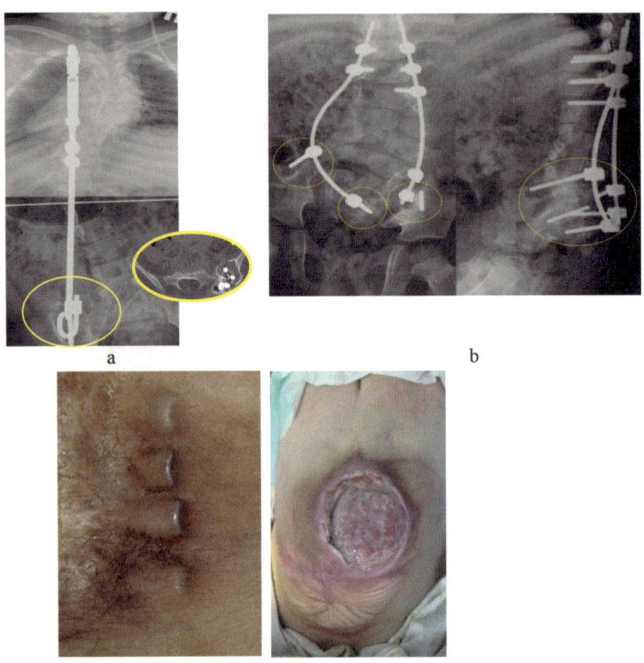

Figure 9.
Complication variants: (a, b) instability of the construction, bone resorbtion; (c) emergence of an "internal pressure sore" due to tissue deficiency; and (d) infection of a pressure sore at the apex of kyphosis.

- Severe, decompensated comorbidities, including genetic disorders and congenital malformations that impose significant limitations on the anticipated lifespan.

- Concurrent brain pathology coupled with profound cognitive impairment and/or recurrent episodes of convulsive seizures.

- Ongoing infectious processes. See **Table 4**.

9. Treatment of segmental spinal dysgenesis

Segmental Spinal Dysgenesis (SSD) is a rare congenital spinal anomaly characterized by localized malformations in the spine's development. It primarily affects the thoracolumbar region and is often accompanied by neurological deficits. SSD involves incomplete formation or absence of vertebral structures, often leading to varying degrees of spinal cord tethering.

The etiology of SSD remains unclear, with theories encompassing vascular disruption, mechanical stress, and teratogenic influences during embryogenesis. Clinical manifestations vary widely, including spinal deformities, neurological deficits, and musculoskeletal abnormalities. SSD can be diagnosed through radiographic imaging and MRI scans, which reveal vertebral abnormalities and associated spinal cord changes [51].

Surgical intervention is often considered to address neurological deficits and prevent deformity progression. However, SSD poses challenges due to the complex anatomical alterations. Long-term outcomes vary, and multidisciplinary management involving orthopedic surgeons, neurosurgeons, and rehabilitation specialists is crucial for optimizing patient care.

The main principle of treatment of SSD involves the removal of rudimentary vertebral elements at the level of dysgenesis, spinal mobilization, posterior instrumental fixation, and anterior spondylodesis (**Figure 2**) [52].

10. Surgical treatment of sacral agenesis

Sacral agenesis is a rare congenital anomaly characterized by the incomplete or absent development of the sacrum, a crucial component of the spine and pelvic structure. This condition arises during embryonic development, often leading to a range of musculoskeletal, neurological, and genitourinary complications. Sacral agenesis may present as a spectrum of severity, with partial agenesis involving varying degrees of sacral vertebrae absence.

Clinically significant forms of sacral agenesis include lumbo-sacral agenesis (**Figure 3**), complete sacral agenesis, and hemisacrum. Lower sacral agenesis (below S1) typically does not require surgical treatment.

11. Conclusions

Progressive spinal deformities are prevalent among patients with open NTDs. The underlying causes of these deformities stem from disturbances in neuromuscular functions and abnormalities in vertebral development. Spinal deformities linked with open NTDs can be broadly categorized into two main groups: predominantly neuromuscular kyphoscoliosis or lordoscoliosis, and severe rigid kyphosis or sharp-angled kyphosis. While kyphoscoliosis is frequently observed in patients with thoracolumbar myelodysplasia, lordoscoliosis is more prevalent in those with low form of MMC.

Timely surgical correction plays a pivotal role in restoring body balance and improving the overall quality of life, thereby mitigating the need for aggressive surgical interventions. The dual growing rod technique offers a safe and effective option for moderate neuromuscular kyphoscoliosis or lordoscoliosis in young patients. Kyphectomy, though challenging and linked to significant complication rates, remains a vital intervention for patients with substantial rigid kyphosis when alternative procedures are limited.

Surgical indications span a spectrum of therapeutic, social, and functional factors. These include preventing and treating pressure sores at the apex of kyphosis, facilitating child care, and ensuring stable positioning during verticalization. The intricacies of spinal pathology within the realm of spinal dysraphia syndrome necessitate personalized surgical planning and the collaboration of a multidisciplinary team. Individualized correction methods, often planned in stages, need to factor in the elevated risk of complications stemming from the diverse range of spinal anomalies.

Author details

Sergey O. Ryabykh[1,2]*, Olga M. Sergeenko[3], Alexander V. Gubin[2], Ilkhom E. Khujanazarov[4,5], Vladimir S. Klimov[1], Dmitry Y. Zinenko[1], Alexey A. Kalashnikov[1], Evgenia M. Berdichevskaya[1] and Timur A. Dzhumatov[2]

1 Veltischev Research and Clinical Institute for Pediatrics and Pediatric Surgery of the Pirogov Russian National Research Medical University, Russian Federation

2 St. Petersburg State University Hospital, Russian Federation

3 National Ilizarov Medical Research Center for Traumatology and Orthopedics, Russian Federation

4 Department of Traumatology, Orthopedics and Neurosurgery, Tashkent Medical Academy, Tashkent, Republic of Uzbekistan

5 Orthopedics and Rehabilitation Department, Republican Specialized Scientific and Practical Medical Center of Traumatology and Orthopedics, Tashkent, Republic of Uzbekistan

*Address all correspondence to: rso_@mail.ru

References

[1] Tortori-Donati P, Rossi A, Cama A. Spinal dysraphism: A review of neuroradiological features with embryological correlations and proposal for a new classification. Neuroradiology. 2000;**42**:471-491

[2] Morota N, Sakamoto H. Surgery for spina bifida occulta: Spinal lipoma and tethered spinal cord. Child's Nervous System. 2023;**10**:2847-2864. DOI: 10.1007/s00381-023-06024-w

[3] Cohen E et al. Patterns and costs of health care use of children with medical complexity. Pediatrics. 2012;**130**(6):e1463-e1470

[4] Eubanks JD, Cheruvu VK. Prevelance of sacral spina bifida occulta and its relationship to age, sex, race, and the sacral table angle: An anatomic osteologic study of three thousand one hundred specimens. Spine. 2009;**15**:1539-1543

[5] Lee JY, Kim JW, Shim Y, Kim SP, Kim KH, Yang J, et al. Myelomeningocele as an anomaly of secondary neurulation. Child's Nervous System. 2022;**38**(11):2091-2099. DOI: 10.1007/s00381-022-05591-8. Epub 2022 Jul 12. Erratum in: Childs Nerv Syst. 2023 Feb;39(2):561-562

[6] Müller EB, Nordwall A. Prevalence of scoliosis in children with myelomeningocele in Western Sweden. Spine (Phila Pa 1976). 1992;**17**:1097-1102

[7] Blount JP, George TM, Koueik J, Iskandar BJ. Concepts in the neurosurgical care of patients with spinal neural tube defects: An embryologic approach. Birth Defects Research. 2019;**111**(19):1564-1576. DOI: 10.1002/bdr2.1588. Epub 2019 Oct 2

[8] Lindseth RE. Myelomeningocele spine. The Pediatric Spine: Principles and Practice. 1994;**2**:1043-1067

[9] Siegel MJ. Ultrassonografia Pediatrica/ Guanabara Koogan. 3rd ed. Brazil: Rio de Janeiro; 2003

[10] McDonnell GV, McCann JP. Issues of medical management in adults with spina bifida. Child's Nervous System. 2000;**16**:222-227

[11] Trivedi J, Thomson JD, Slakey JB, Banta JV, Jones PW. Clinical and radiographic predictors of scoliosis in patients with myelomeningocele. The Journal of Bone and Joint Surgery. American Volume. 2002;**84-A**:1389-1394

[12] Kayaba H, Hebiguchi T, Itoh Y, Yoshino H, Mizuno M, Morii M, et al. Evaluation of anorectal function in patients with tethered cord syndrome: Saline enema test and fecoflowmetry. Journal of Neurosurgery: Spine. 2003;**98**(3):251-257

[13] Yamada S, Won DJ, Yamada SM. Pathophysiology of tethered cord syndrome: Correlation with symptomatology. Neurosurgical Focus. 2004;**16**(2):1-5

[14] Duddy JC, Caird J, Connolly P. Repair of a large thoracolumbar myelomeningocele with associated lumbar kyphosis. Acta Neurochirurgica. 2013;**155**:1965-1968

[15] Dunn RN, Bomela LN. Kyphectomy in children with severe myelomeningocele-related kyphosis. Spine Deform. 2016;**4**:230-236

[16] Schroeder JE, Barzilay Y, Hasharoni A, Kaplan L. Long-term

outcome of surgical correction of congenital kyphosis in patients with myelomeningocele (MMC) with segmental spino-pelvic fixation. Evidence-Based Spine-Care Journal. 2011;**2**:17-22

[17] Eysel P et al. Development of scoliosis in myelomeningocele. Differences in the history caused by idiopathic pattern. Neurosurgical Review. 1993;**16**(4):301-306

[18] Guille JT et al. Congenital and developmental deformities of the spine in children with myelomeningocele. Journal of the American Academy of Orthopaedic Surgeons. 2006;**14**(5):294-302

[19] Carstens C et al. Development of pathological lumbar kyphosis in myelomeningocele. Bone & Joint Journal. 1996;**78**(6):945-950

[20] Park TS et al. Progressive spasticity and scoliosis in children with myelomeningocele: Radiological investigation and surgical treatment. Journal of Neurosurgery. 1985;**62**(3): 367-375

[21] Ryabykh SO, Pavlova OM, Savin DM, Burcev AV, Gubin AV. Surgical management of myelomeningocelerelated spinal deformities. World Neurosurgery. 2018;**112**:e431-e441. DOI: 10.1016/j.wneu.2018.01.058

[22] Ko AL, Song K, Ellenbogen RG, Avellino AM. Retrospective review of multilevel spinal fusion combined with spinal cord transection for treatment of kyphoscoliosis in pediatric myelomeningocele patients. Spine (Phila Pa 1976). 2007;32:2493-2501

[23] Parisini P et al. Surgical treatment of scoliosis in myelomeningocele. Studies in Health Technology and Informatics. 2001;**91**:442-447

[24] Tachdijian M. Myelomeningocele/scoliosis. In: Pediatric Orthopaedics. Philadelphia: WB Saunders; 1990. pp. 1843-1848

[25] Müller EB, Nordwall A, Odén A. Progression of scoliosis in children with myelomeningocele. Spine. 1994;**19**(2):147-150

[26] Hudgins RJ, Gilreath CL. Tethered spinal cord following repair of myelomeningocele. Neurosurgical Focus. 2004;**16**(2):1-4

[27] Herman JM et al. Analysis of 153 patients with myelomeningocele or spinal lipoma reoperated upon for a tethered cord. Pediatric Neurosurgery. 1993;**19**(5):243-249

[28] Sarwark JF et al. Tethered cord syndrome in low motor level children with myelomeningocele. Pediatric Neurosurgery. 1996;**25**(6):295-301

[29] Bowman RM et al. Tethered cord release: A long-term study in 114 patients: Clinical article. Journal of Neurosurgery: Pediatrics. 2009;**3**(3):181-187

[30] Dias MS. Neurosurgical causes of scoliosis in patients with myelomeningocele: An evidence-based literature review. Journal of Neurosurgery: Pediatrics. 2005;**103**(1):24-35

[31] Samuelsson L, Skoog M. Ambulation in patients with myelomeningocele: A multivariate statistical analysis. Journal of Pediatric Orthopaedics. 1988;**8**(5):569-575

[32] Sharma S et al. Prevalence of complications in neuromuscular scoliosis

surgery: A literature meta-analysis from the past 15 years. European Spine Journal. 2013;**22**(6):1230-1249

[33] Wai EK et al. Assessing physical disability in children with spina bifida and scoliosis. Journal of Pediatric Orthopaedics. 2000;**20**(6):765-770

[34] Wai EK et al. The relationship between function, self-perception, and spinal deformity: Implications for treatment of scoliosis in children with spina bifida. Journal of Pediatric Orthopaedics. 2005;**25**(1):64-69

[35] Feng F, Tan H, Li X, Chen C, Li Z, Zhang J, et al. Radiographic characteristics in congenital scoliosis associated with split cord malformation: A retrospective study of 266 surgical cases. BMC Musculoskeletal Disorders. 2017;**18**(1):420. DOI: 10.1186/s12891-017-1782-z

[36] Sergeenko (Pavlova) OM, Savin DM, Ryabykh SO. Treatment of spinal deformity with diastematomyelia type I: One-stage, two-stage surgery and new technique (vertebral column resection through wide bony septum). Child's Nervous System. 2022;**38**(1):163-172. DOI: 10.1007/s00381-021-05382-7

[37] Sato T, Yonezawa I, Onda S, Yoshikawa K, Takano H, Shimamura Y, et al. Surgical treatment for lumbar hyperlordosis after resection of a spinal lipoma associated with spina bifida: A case report. Medicine (Baltimore). 2017;**96**:e7895

[38] Bas CE, Preminger J, Olgun ZD, Demirkiran G, Sponseller P, Yazici M. Safety and efficacy of apical resection following growth-friendly instrumentation in myelomeningocele patients with gibbus: Growing rod versus Luque trolley. Journal of Pediatric Orthopedics. 2015;**35**:e98-e103

[39] Yuan N et al. The effect of scoliosis surgery on lung function in the immediate postoperative period. Spine. 2005;**30**(19):2182-2185

[40] Samdani AF et al. A patient with myelomeningocele: Is untethering necessary prior to scoliosis correction? Neurosurgical Focus. 2010;**29**(1):E8

[41] Wild A et al. Is sacral instrumentation mandatory to address pelvic obliquity in neuromuscular thoracolumbar scoliosis due to myelomeningocele? Spine. 2001;**26**(14):E325-E329

[42] Rodgers WB et al. Spinal deformity in myelodysplasia: Correction with posterior pedicle screw instrumentation. Spine. 1997;**22**(20):2435-2443

[43] Guille JT et al. The feasibility, safety, and utility of vertebral wedge osteotomies for the fusionless treatment of paralytic scoliosis. Spine. 2003;**28**(20S):S266-S274

[44] Cardoso M, Keating RF. Neurosurgical management of spinal dysraphism and neurogenic scoliosis. Spine. 2009;**34**(17):1775-1782

[45] Karami M, Akbarnia BA. Ilizarov kyphectomy technique in the management of the gibbus deformity with an open wound in meningomyelocele patients: A case report with five years of follow-up. European Spine Journal. 2022;**31**:3713-3718. DOI: 10.1007/s00586-021-07058-x

[46] Smith JT, Novais E. Treatment of gibbus deformity associated with myelomeningocele in the young child with use of the vertical expandable prosthetic titanium rib (VEPTR). The Journal of Bone and Joint Surgery. American Volume. 2010;**92**(12):2211-2215

[47] Drummond DS, Moreau M, Cruess RL. The results and complications of surgery for the paralytic hip and spine in myelomeningocele. Bone & Joint Journal. 1980;**62**(1):49-53

[48] Hatlen T et al. Contributory factors to postoperative spinal fusion complications for children with myelomeningocele. Spine. 2010;**35**(13):1294-1299

[49] Sponseller PD et al. Deep wound infections after neuromuscular scoliosis surgery: A multicenter study of risk factors and treatment outcomes. Spine. 2000;**25**(19):2461-2466

[50] Boemers TML et al. Urological problems after surgical treatment of scoliosis in children with myelomeningocele. The Journal of urology. 1996;**155**(3):1066-1069

[51] Faciszewski T, Winter RB, Lonstein JE, Sane S, Erickson D. Segmental spinal dysgenesis. A disorder different from spinal agenesis. JBJS. 1995;**77**(4):530-537

[52] Pavlova OM, Ryabykh SO, Kozyrev DA, Gubin AV. Surgical treatment of thoracolumbar segmental spinal dysgenesis: Optimal type of fusion. World Neurosurgery. 2017;**106**:551-556. DOI: 10.1016/j.wneu.2017.07.031

Chapter 7

Advances in Early Onset Scoliosis Management: A Narrative Review of Treatment Modalities

Hossein Nematian, Andrew Clarke, Zahra Vahdati, Mohammad Hossein Nabian and Saeed Reza Mehrpour

Abstract

Early-onset scoliosis (EOS) refers to a heterogeneous group of spinal deformities in children aged below 10 years. These conditions exhibit significant variations in their causes, natural progression, and available treatment options. As EOS progresses, it can lead to thoracic insufficiency syndrome, characterized by an altered thoracic structure that hinders normal respiratory function and lung development. This chapter provides an overview of the current treatment methods for EOS, focusing on nonoperative interventions, growth-friendly surgical techniques, and advanced technologies. Nonoperative approaches include bracing, casting, and physiotherapy, aiming to slow or halt curve progression. Surgical interventions are often necessary for severe cases and utilize growth-friendly techniques such as traditional or magnetically controlled growing rods. This chapter highlights the various treatment options available for EOS, emphasizing the importance of early detection and intervention. By effectively managing EOS, healthcare professionals can optimize patient outcomes, minimize complications, and improve the quality of life for affected children. Potential avenues for future research and advancements in EOS treatment are discussed, focusing on minimizing complications and maximizing functional outcomes for affected children. Furthermore, this chapter aims to guide healthcare professionals in making informed decisions regarding the management of EOS.

Keywords: early-onset scoliosis, growth-friendly surgery, techniques, conservative treatment, complications, outcomes, quality of life

1. Introduction

Early-onset Scoliosis (EOS) encompasses a spectrum of spinal pathologies that arise during the growth phase, presenting in diverse forms. The intrinsic complexity of EOS has posed challenges in formulating a comprehensive and universally accepted definition, thereby affecting the consensus on diagnosis and management within the orthopedic community. The term EOS was first introduced by Ponseti and Friedman to characterize idiopathic scoliosis in patients under 10 years old [1]. Their observations highlighted a notably less favorable prognosis for these younger patients compared to their older counterparts. Subsequently, in 1954, James further refined the classification of idiopathic scoliosis, categorizing it into three distinct age-based groups: infantile (≤3 years), juvenile (4–9 years), and adolescent (10 years to skeletal maturity) [2]. However, Dickson raised concerns regarding the classification of juvenile idiopathic scoliosis, suggesting an overlap with the infantile subgroup [3]. In later years, Dickson proposed a subdivision of idiopathic scoliosis into early-onset (0–5 years) and late-onset (>5 years) categories [4]. It is noteworthy that despite the recent adoption of this classification in the literature, it has been acknowledged that the treatment approaches for children aged 5–10 years more closely resemble those employed for children under 5 years of age rather than those for children over 10 years of age. Consequently, the Growing Spine Study Group (GSSG) and the Children Spine Study Group (CSSG) defined EOS as any spinal deformity present before the age of 10 years, irrespective of its underlying cause [5, 6]. In 2014, a research team led by Vitale proposed a comprehensive definition for EOS that incorporates both age of onset and etiology. They categorized EOS into four distinct etiological groups: idiopathic, neuromuscular, congenital, and syndromic [6]. This multifaceted approach aimed to enhance the understanding and classification of EOS, thereby facilitating more precise diagnosis and tailored management strategies.

EOS is characterized by a rapid progression, underscoring the importance of expeditious clinical diagnosis and timely referral to a specialized pediatric orthopedic unit [6]. Extensive research has consistently demonstrated that the timing of EOS onset significantly influences the eventual curvature severity and prognosis, with earlier onset correlating with more adverse outcomes [7]. Furthermore, untreated EOS often culminates in substantial spinal deformities, ultimately resulting in a shortened spine, linked to heightened mortality rates and cardiopulmonary compromise [8, 9]. Historically, Scott et al. reported a linear progression rate of approximately 5° per year in EOS cases, highlighting the aggressive nature of the condition [7]. Subsequent investigations by Pehrsson et al. have elucidated the increased risk of severe scoliosis development in patients with early-onset EOS, juxtaposed with adolescent-onset scoliosis, further underscoring the significance of prompt intervention [8]. This elevated morbidity and mortality risk among early-onset EOS patients can be attributed to structural alterations constraining the thoracic cavity, leading to restrictive lung disease, cardiovascular complications, and respiratory failure [10]. Consequently, a comprehensive assessment of EOS should explore the intricate interplay between lung, spine, and thorax development. This holistic approach is imperative for a thorough understanding of EOS's deleterious impact on cardiopulmonary function and underscores the necessity for timely clinical intervention to mitigate its adverse consequences.

The consideration of lung development plays a pivotal role in comprehending EOS's historical and progressive aspects within the context of orthopedics. The intricate interplay between the growth of the thoracic cage, spine, and lungs has been extensively explored in existing academic literature. In humans, the skeletal system undergoes two distinct phases of rapid growth, the initial one transpiring from birth to 5 years of age and the subsequent phase occurring during puberty [11, 12]. Concomitantly, lung development exhibits a nonlinear trajectory, characterized by alveolar-capillary proliferation peaking around birth and reaching completion by the age of 2 years, with a cessation phase extending until the age of 8 years. Simultaneously, the bronchial tree's volume undergoes augmentation with the child's growth [13]. Consequently, any disruption within the growth dynamics of the thoracic cage-spinal complex can exert detrimental effects on alveolar number and volume as well as the overall lung growth. The simultaneous progression of spinal deformities attributable to EOS during the critical phase of pulmonary alveolar development can significantly impair pulmonary function [9, 14]. Notably, instances of lung hypoplasia, marked by diminished alveoli and arteries, have been observed in patients whose scoliosis becomes pronounced during this crucial period of lung growth, often accompanied by emphysematous alterations [15]. Furthermore, Karol et al. have elucidated a direct correlation between thoracic height and pulmonary function, establishing that a shorter thoracic spine is associated with reduced forced vital capacity (FVC) and an increased propensity for restrictive pulmonary disease. Their research highlights that, in order to avert severe restrictive lung disease (FVC < 50%), the thoracic height should measure greater than 22 cm at skeletal maturity [9]. However, Johnston et al. conducted a study to assess the relationship between pulmonary function and thoracic spine height in EOS patients who underwent corrective surgery. The study revealed that, regardless of whether the patients had a thoracic height of 18 cm or more, their pulmonary function was significantly compromised if they had residual curves exceeding 50°. This raised questions about the validity of using a fixed threshold such as 18 cm as an EOS outcome parameter [16]. The expanding understanding of lung growth dynamics and the long-term consequences of early spinal fusion in scoliosis have influenced current clinical practice. Consequently, spinal fusion procedures before the age of 8 years are now not preferred, with a preference for postponing surgery until the age of 10 years to optimize patient outcomes [17]. These findings underscore the critical role of interdisciplinary collaboration between orthopedic and pulmonary specialists in managing EOS and emphasize the importance of informed clinical decision-making based on the latest scientific insights.

The management of severe scoliosis in skeletally mature adolescents predominantly revolves around spinal fusion, a procedure known to entail the sacrifice of spinal mobility and potential impediments to longitudinal growth. Conversely, addressing severe scoliosis in pediatric patients presents a constellation of distinctive challenges, underscored by the ongoing maturation of the spine, thoracic cavity, and cardiopulmonary system, often complicated by the presence of intricate functional, cognitive, or medical comorbidities. Treatment of EOS assumes paramount importance with multifaceted goals, encompassing the arrest of progression or correction of deformity, the preservation of spinal growth, the optimization of thoracic capacity, and the enhancement of pulmonary function. These objectives are fundamentally directed toward averting cardiopulmonary compromise and optimizing the health-related quality of life [18]. The knowledge derived from extensive research elucidates the intricate interplay between the chest wall, lungs, and spinal column. This deep understanding has directed therapeutic approaches toward cultivating a well-developed thoracic cavity, augmentation of lung volume, and refinement of pulmonary function [9, 14]. Thus, a shift toward growth-friendly treatments has emerged. The therapeutic spectrum for EOS spans both nonoperative interventions and surgical approaches. While nonoperative methods, notably corrective casting and bracing, play a pivotal role in forestalling or delaying the need for spinal surgery and should be considered the cornerstone of treatment, it is essential to acknowledge their inherent limitations. In rapidly progressing curvature that necessitates surgical stabilization, innovative “growth-friendly” corrective techniques have emerged as an indispensable resource within the therapeutic arsenal.

2. Nonoperative treatment

The nonoperative management of spinal deformities encompasses a range of therapeutic modalities, such as bracing, casting, halo-gravity traction (HGT), and physiotherapy, which have demonstrated a potential for achieving favorable correction outcomes in select patient populations. These interventions often serve a dual purpose of achieving satisfactory correction and postponing the need for surgical intervention, making them valuable components of comprehensive treatment strategies. HGT frequently assumes an adjunctive role in the therapeutic landscape, commonly complementing other treatments including surgical interventions [19, 20]. Its applicability is particularly indicated for patients presenting with severe and inflexible spinal curves, those afflicted by scoliosis accompanied by kyphosis, and individuals experiencing compromised pulmonary or nutritional status. The role of physiotherapy in managing idiopathic scoliosis in skeletally immature children remains a topic of ongoing debate and necessitates further substantiation through rigorous validation studies [21]. Casting and bracing are considered two major nonoperative interventions for spinal deformity.

2.1 Casting

Serial casting represents a highly effective conservative approach to managing EOS, which can help preserve growth potential and potentially obviate the need for surgical intervention, particularly in cases of idiopathic scoliosis [22, 23]. The specific techniques employed in serial casting can vary across different studies. Typically, patients receive general anesthesia, followed by applying traction and padding placement on prominent bony areas. Subsequently, plaster is used and shaped with derotational forces to address scoliosis. Casts are scheduled for replacement every 2 to 3 months, with regular clinical and radiological evaluations to accommodate the rapid growth phase of the spine and trunk, tailored to each patient's growth trajectory.

Serial casting is generally recommended when the curvature exceeds 25°, shows a minimum documented progression of 10°, or exhibits a rib-vertebral angle difference greater than 20° [24]. Early initiation of casting has demonstrated the ability to halt the progression and even correct EOS, yielding a durable and stable outcome in otherwise healthy children [25]. Therefore, the commencement of serial casting should occur as early as possible, as older age and more significant curvature have been identified as potential risk factors for unsuccessful casting treatments [26, 27].

In a study conducted by Gussous et al. [26], 74 consecutive patients were treated with casting therapy, comprising 41 with idiopathic scoliosis and 33 with non-idiopathic scoliosis. Their average age was 19 months, and they were followed up for an average of 11 months. The results revealed that in the idiopathic group, the Cobb angle was successfully corrected from 47° to 27°, whereas in the nonidiopathic group, it improved from 62° to 57°. Notably, the idiopathic group exhibited a higher correction rate compared to the nonidiopathic group. During the final follow-up, minor complications were observed in 8% of cases, including issues such as pressure sores, pyogenic granuloma, exacerbations of gastroesophageal reflux, and humeral fractures, which were attributed to cast-related impaction by parents. Major complications occurred in 4% of cases, including subclavian vein thrombosis, cardiac arrest during general anesthesia induction, and a tragic death due to an acute asthma attack. The study findings suggest that individuals with idiopathic scoliosis, characterized by greater flexibility and milder curvature, tend to respond more favorably to casting treatment compared to those with non-idiopathic scoliosis. Moreover, progressive idiopathic scoliosis patients achieved superior curve correction with casting compared to nonidiopathic scoliosis patients. Commencing casting before 24 months led to improved curve correction outcomes. Patients who ultimately required surgery are typically presented at an older age with a higher Cobb angle than those who transitioned to thoracolumbosacral orthosis (TLSO) treatment. Although rib-vertebral angle difference (RVAD) predicts progression in infantile idiopathic scoliosis, it did not demonstrate predictive values in response to casting for either the idiopathic or nonidiopathic scoliosis groups.

In recent times, there has been a resurgence of interest in the previously abandoned Mehta casting technique for EOS treatment. Mehta's approach, as described in his 2005 paper [25], aimed to utilize casting to harness the growth potential in EOS and correct progressive curves that could otherwise lead to severe deformities. This method involves meticulously applying a plaster jacket on a Cotrel frame, incorporating a head halter and pelvic traction, known as elongation-derotation-flexion casting. This approach applies a three-dimensional correction force to counteract scoliotic deformity.

Mehta's groundbreaking study involved 136 children under 4 years with progressive infantile scoliosis (diagnosed before age 3 years). Among the 94 children who received early referral at an average age of 1 year and 7 months, with an average Cobb angle of 32° (ranging from 11° to 65°), their scoliosis resolved by the mean age of 3.5 years, obviating the need for further treatment, allowing them to lead normal lives. In contrast, among the 42 children with a late referral at an average age of 2.5 years and a mean Cobb angle of 52° (ranging from 23° to 92°), casting was ineffective in reversing the deformity, leading to spinal fusion in 36% of these cases.

It's worth noting that the nonidiopathic population did not exhibit the same promising results in significantly reducing morphologic deformity; however, it did delay the need for surgical intervention [28]. Nonetheless, if young patients can tolerate the associated complications, casting remains a viable and effective treatment option for EOS.

2.2 Bracing

The effectiveness of bracing in treating adolescent idiopathic scoliosis has yielded promising results, particularly for patients with curves ranging from 25 to 40° [29, 30].

However, the use of bracing for EOS remains a topic of debate, with limited research available [31–33].

Recent investigations by Thometz et al. have shown encouraging outcomes when employing an elongation-bending-derotation brace (EBDB) in children with infantile or juvenile scoliosis, including neuromuscular, congenital, and idiopathic cases [31, 32]. During a 12-month follow-up, the juvenile group exhibited a 25.7% curve correction and 42.9% stabilization, whereas the infantile group showed a remarkable 50% curve correction and 32.1% stabilization. Notably, no patients required surgery during this follow-up period. Additionally, the authors focused on nine infants with idiopathic scoliosis (average age: 11 months) treated with EBDB for a minimum of 2 years. Four patients achieved complete correction with bracing alone (final curve ≤10°), whereas five patients with more rigid curves demonstrated improvement from an average of 57° to 21°.

However, it is important to acknowledge the relatively short follow-up duration and the absence of a second growth spurt assessment in these studies [31, 32]. While bracing offers convenience by allowing removal as needed, casting provides continuous corrective force because it cannot be removed. While bracing may be an effective treatment option for EOS, further research is required to directly compare the efficacy of bracing versus casting in this patient population.

3. Operative treatment

Performing long spinal fusion procedures in patients with early-onset scoliosis (EOS) can pose risks to thoracic growth and pulmonary function. It may increase the likelihood of complications such as the crankshaft phenomenon or decompensation.

However, the introduction of growth-sparing spinal surgery has revolutionized the management of EOS patients. These innovative surgical approaches can correct severe spinal deformities while preserving the potential for thoracic cage and spinal complex growth until the child nears skeletal maturity [34]. The primary objective of these nonfusion surgical techniques is to achieve the appropriate spine length, specifically a T1–T12 length of at least 18 cm at the time of skeletal maturation. This achievement provides access to approximately 45% of normal lung volume (vital capacity) and helps mitigate the long-term repercussions associated with traditional spinal fusion procedures [9].

There is remarkably little information in the literature depicting the impact of these newer expandable devices on lung function in children with EOS after the initial implantation, during expansion, and after spine fusion—no randomized controlled trials state whose devices and surgical strategies provide the greatest respiratory benefit to patients. In addition, most series describing preoperative and postoperative changes in lung function among children with EOS include small numbers of subjects [3, 7, 25]. Most reports have studied children receiving vertical expandable prosthetic titanium ribs but not other growth-sparing or modulating devices [25–27].

Growth-friendly surgical techniques for EOS were classified by Skaggs et al. based on the applied correction force [35]. These techniques fall into three categories:

1. Distraction-based implants encompass traditional growing rods (TGR), vertical expandable prosthetic titanium rib (VEPTR), and magnetically controlled growing rod (MCGR). This approach applies mechanical distractive forces to the spine segments, ribs, and/or pelvis.

2. Compression-based implants include vertebral body stapling (VBS) and vertebral body tethers (VBT). This method involves applying a compressive force to the convex side of the deformity, resulting in growth inhibition on the ipsilateral side.

3. Guided growth systems, such as the Luque Trolley and Shilla techniques, anchor the end and apical vertebrae, allowing the spine to slide along the rod.

While growth-friendly surgeries maintain growth potential in EOS patients, they come with a high complication rate, extended treatment duration, and additional costs.

3.1 Distraction-based systems

3.1.1 Traditional growing rods

Traditional growing rods (TGRs) are the preferred technique and are considered the standard of care for treating EOS characterized by long curves [36]. These rods achieve correction through distraction and maintain it through proximal and distal instrumentation and fusion. This approach preserves growth potential, particularly lung growth, by leaving spine segments unfused and allowing for lengthening procedures. The concept of using rods for distraction to correct scoliosis, as an alternative to spinal fusion, was initially introduced by Harrington [37]. Subsequently, Moe et al. attempted a modification with a "subcutaneous rod" technique, but it yielded unsatisfactory results and a high rate of complications [38, 39]. Akbarnia et al. later demonstrated improved outcomes by implementing the dual-growing rod technique over a single rod [40]. While there is a consensus that growing-rod surgery is primarily indicated when bracing or casting treatments fail and the curvature exceeds 60° in patients younger than 10 years old, theoretically, TGRs can be considered for any patient with ongoing skeletal immaturity [41].

Performing TGR surgeries involves a series of procedures under general anesthesia every 6 months to lengthen the rod throughout a child's development. Unfortunately, this technique comes with a substantial risk of complications, often necessitating unplanned surgeries for management. These complications encompass rod fracture, anchor failure, deep surgical site infections, repeated exposure to anesthesia, neurological issues, proximal junctional kyphosis, and prolonged postoperative recovery. Moreover, this method carries both direct and indirect financial burdens for families and the healthcare system, making it a significant concern in its application [42, 43]. Multiple studies have reported a high rate of complications, with as many as 77% of patients experiencing at least one complication [40, 42, 44, 45]. Notably, the reported complication rates can vary due to differences in fixation methods, types of growing rods, and surgical strategies [46, 47]. This variation has led to ongoing controversy regarding the ideal approach for TGR surgeries.

Several well-recognized risk factors contribute to complications associated with growing rods, including younger age at the initial surgery, using a single rod, longer lengthening intervals, thoracic hyperkyphosis, and the placement of rods subcutaneously. The elevated incidence of complications in treating EOS with traditional growing rods (TGRs) can be attributed to the extended treatment duration, primarily due to the young age of patients when the initial rod placement occurs and the substantial number of surgical procedures needed throughout the treatment period. Research has demonstrated that the likelihood of complications increases by 24% for each additional surgical procedure. Additionally, for every year following surgery, complications decreased by 13% [42].

In a 2010 study by Bess et al. [42], the effects of TGRs were compared in 140 children with EOS. Participants were divided into two groups based on the type of growing rods used, with 51% receiving single TGRs and 49% receiving dual TGRs. Among the 140 participants, 81 experienced at least one complication, resulting in a 57% complication rate. For those using single TGRs, this rate was slightly higher at 60.6%. A total of 177 episodes of complications were observed, with 94 occurring in 43 participants in the single TGRs group and 83 in 38 participants in the dual TGRs group. Among these complications, 74 necessitated unplanned surgeries for management (41.8%), with 42 occurring in participants with single TGRs (46.7%) and 32 in participants with dual TGRs (38.5%). However, statistically, none of these differences were significant. Interestingly, the study revealed that the use of dual TGRs, compared to single TGRs, was associated with a lower risk of implant-related complications and a reduced likelihood of hook dislodgments and unplanned implant-related surgeries ($P \leq .05$).

While previous literature has highlighted the superiority and cost-effectiveness of dual TGRs [48, 49], it is important to acknowledge that using dual TGRs may not always be a feasible or preferred option. Factors such as patient size, the amount of supporting soft tissue, and the nature of the spinal deformity can limit their applicability.

In a 2021 study by Luhmann et al., it was demonstrated that the use of single-growing rod structures, particularly in children aged 4–8 years, can yield acceptable outcomes for EOS patients, especially when dual rods are not considered feasible due to factors such as curve rotation, magnitude, kyphosis, and inadequate soft tissue coverage for a convex spinal rod. The study suggests that single TGRs and MCGRs can serve as bridging treatments for patients aged 3–7 years with low body weight and short T1–T12 distances. These rods can be employed until the patient attains the necessary weight and height growth, at this point, the surgical construct can be converted to dual TGRs or MCGRs [50].

Nematian et al. [45] conducted a study involving 35 cases of EOS treated with single TGR insertion, encompassing 162 lengthening episodes and 42 unplanned surgeries. Their findings revealed that a substantial 77.1% of patients encountered at least one complication during the course of treatment. The mean preoperative Cobb angle for the major curve was 59.2° ± 5.8°, and this was corrected to 38.2° ± 6.0° at the final follow-up, demonstrating a significant improvement ($P < .001$). However, no statistically significant difference was noted in pre- and postoperative T1–T12 kyphosis measurements. It is worth noting that the relatively higher complication rate observed in this study, compared to previous literature, could be attributed to the nature of the study population. Case selection in this study was not random, and the children treated were of low socio-economic status, referred late, and tended to have more complicated conditions. The study's conclusions suggest that even when dual TGRs are not feasible or preferred due to the patient's physical condition and the specific characteristics of the deformity, the use of single TGRs should be minimized. Conservative treatments and early fusion are recommended as alternatives. The long-term results and complications associated with single TGRs indicate that their disadvantages may outweigh their advantages even when used as a bridge treatment. To reduce the incidence of complications in growing rod treatment, the study recommends personalized treatment plans based on the etiology of EOS and the patient's physical condition (including age, respiratory status, and degree of deformity). Delaying treatment initiation based on the rate of progression, utilizing dual rods with appropriate diameters, and employing screws as anchors in sufficient numbers to secure foundation sites whenever feasible are also suggested strategies.

In conclusion, while TGRs remain the standard for EOS treatment, dual TGRs are preferred, but patient-specific factors may limit their use. MCGRs offer convenience but introduce unique risks. Single TGRs should be used cautiously, with alternative treatments considered when appropriate. Personalized treatment and careful patient selection are crucial for minimizing complications.

3.1.2 Magnetically controlled growing rods

In 2015, the FDA granted approval for the use of MCGR in treating EOS [36]. MCGR represents a more recent method of distraction surgery designed to address the issues associated with TGR. MCGR incorporates telescopic distraction actuators within each rod, and these actuators can be magnetically adjusted externally using a remote control for lengthening, eliminating the need for repeated surgeries. Surgical placement and fixation of the rods using screws or hooks are similar to TGR constructs. Notably, the initial surgery in the MCGR method is the sole planned surgery until the completion of the growing rod treatment [51]. While there is no consensus on the ideal lengthening intervals or number of distractions, most surgeons opt for more frequent rod lengthening compared to TGRs, typically occurring every 3–6 months [52, 53]. Theoretically, the indications for MCGRs should align with those for TGRs; however, MCGRs are not officially approved in all regions.

Akbarnia et al. [53] conducted a study involving 14 EOS patients (mean age: 8 years and 10 months) who received MCGRs, with an average follow-up period of 10 months. The study demonstrated a 50% correction rate after the initial surgery, which was well-maintained at the final follow-up. Additionally, spine height increased from 292 to 322 mm post-surgery and reached 338 mm at the final follow-up. On average, each patient underwent 4.9 distraction procedures. Complications included one case of superficial infection, one instance of a prominent implant, and three losses of initial distraction after the index procedure. The study concluded that MCGRs serve as a viable alternative treatment option, providing comparable results to TGRs but without the anticipated complications. La Rosa et al. [52] reported that MCGRs offer benefits over TGRs by preventing surgical scarring, surgical site infections, and psychological distress typically associated with the multiple surgeries required by TGRs. This reduction in infections and wound healing issues benefits patients and reduces medical costs. Akbarnia et al. [54] also demonstrated that MCGRs achieve similar results to TGRs regarding major curve correction and spinal and thoracic height. MCGRs are proposed to minimize the need for planned surgical interventions by avoiding repeated open lengthening procedures, thereby reducing the risk of complications. However, concerns about unplanned surgical revisions due to complications remain. In addition, Teoh et al. [34] found that, while MCGRs were linked to lower rates of both deep and superficial infections compared to TGRs, they were associated with a significantly increased risk of metalwork problems and unplanned revisions (OR = 4.67). Their study also indicated a higher overall complication rate compared to conventional growing rods [33]. In summary, MCGRs offer advantages in terms of reduced infections and improved patient experience but come with a higher risk of metalwork issues and unplanned revisions. Aslan et al. [55] conducted a study assessing the psychological effects of multiple surgeries on patients' mental health. They found that MCGRs did not improve psychological effects on patient mental health compared to TGRs. Despite the noninvasiveness of the MCGR procedure, it did not yield the anticipated benefits in terms of psychological well-being and health-related quality of life, as compared to TGR [56].

While MCGRs offer the advantage of avoiding repetitive surgical procedures for lengthening, they still share many complications with TGRs and introduce a few novel ones. Coupled with their high cost and limited availability, particularly in developing countries, MCGRs have lost some of their initial appeal. They are now viewed as merely one of several therapeutic options alongside TGR [34, 57]. In conclusion, further research involving larger sample sizes and longer follow-up periods is essential to better understand this relatively new technique and its optimal utilization.

In summary, MCGRs offer advantages in terms of convenience but come with increased risks and psychological outcomes similar to TGRs. Further research with larger sample sizes and longer follow-up periods is needed to better understand and utilize this technique effectively.

3.1.3 Vertical expandable prosthetic titanium rib

VEPTR devices are constructed from titanium alloy longitudinal rods that function as distraction devices. These rods are equipped with anchors placed at the ribs and spine, allowing for the comprehensive management of three-dimensional thoracic deformities, with or without expansion thoracoplasty [58].

VEPTRs were originally developed by Dr. Robert Cambell and Melvin Smith with the primary aim of treating thoracic insufficiency syndrome (TIS) linked to congenital scoliosis and fused ribs [59]. While their main indication is for patients with TIS, they are occasionally employed for individuals with EOS who are at risk of developing secondary TIS [60].

Initial studies exhibited promising results, including Cobb angle corrections, increased lung expansion space, and overall spine growth [59, 61]. However, subsequent research has failed to consistently support these initial findings. A 15-year study by Ramirez et al. [62] revealed that respiratory function did not improve significantly, spine growth was moderate, and Cobb angle correction fell short of expectations. Additionally, VEPTRs have been associated with notable complication rates, with proximal fixation failure being the most common issue. Lengthening of VEPTRs is typically performed every 4–6 months, and the complication rate can be as high as 100%, limiting their widespread application [63].

Studies by Campbell et al. reported complication rates as high as 163% in patients with congenital scoliosis, Hasler et al. documented 100% complication rates in non-congenital scoliosis patients, and Ramirez et al. observed rates as high as 73.1% in neuromuscular scoliosis patients [61, 64, 65]. Consequently, doubts have arisen regarding the benefits of VEPTRs, and when they are considered, there is a consensus to approach their use with caution, favoring a multidisciplinary approach.

In summary, VEPTR devices were initially promising for managing thoracic deformities but have faced challenges with complications and limited benefits in subsequent research. Their use is now approached cautiously, with a preference for multidisciplinary evaluation.

3.2 Compression-based implants

Compression-based implants function by addressing spinal deformities by applying a compressive force to the convex side of the curve, which hinders its growth while allowing the development of the concave side, aligning with the Hueter-Volkmann principle. This principle suggests that physeal growth can be regulated through mechanical compression, promoting growth by reducing mechanical load [66].

However, concerns related to overcorrection of the curve, particularly in immature patients, have been associated with compression-based implants. Consequently, some surgeons recommend reserving this technique for patients with limited remaining growth potential, typically in the 9- to 10-year-old age range [18].

Despite these strict indications and limited applications, the primary advantage of vertical body tethering (VBT) and vertebral body stapling (VBS) is their ability to preserve growth potential and spinal segment mobility. On the downside, these techniques can be associated with surgical approach complications, including pulmonary and bowel issues resulting from anterior surgeries.

As VBS and VBT are relatively recent methods for treating spinal deformities, the available literature is limited. Because of the absence of long-term results and discrepancies in complication rates or adverse events reported in studies, further research is needed to comprehensively assess their effectiveness, safety profile, and the optimal age range for patients to benefit from these techniques.

3.2.1 Vertebral staples techniques

The concept of VBS was initially proposed by Nachlas et al. [67]; however, early attempts showed poor results [68]. In Guille et al. introduced a modern nitinol C-shaped staple that improved compression across the growth plate [69].

VBS entails the placement of metal staples to selectively inhibit spinal growth on the convex side while preserving motion segments throughout the spine without fusion. The procedure involves thoracoscopic stapling for thoracic curves and a mini-open retroperitoneal approach for motion segments below the diaphragm, specifically at the T12–L1 level and below [70, 71].

Traditionally, moderate immature curves have been managed with bracing; however, when bracing is no longer effective, VBS becomes a viable option [30]. The current indications for VBS are quite stringent and include idiopathic scoliosis, a Risser sign of 0–2, a curvature degree ranging from 25° to 40°, and failure of brace treatment [72].

Cahill et al. conducted a review involving 63 patients who underwent VBS at a mean age of 10.78 years, with a mean follow-up duration of 3.62 years. Their findings demonstrated the effectiveness of VBS in preventing progression and fusion in thoracic and lumbar curves with mean Cobb angles of 29.5° and 31.1°, respectively. Seventy-four percent of patients with thoracic VBS and eighty-two percent of those with lumbar VBS did not exhibit progression and/or fusion [73].

In summary, VBS has evolved with modern techniques and has shown promise in managing scoliosis in select patient populations, particularly when bracing is no longer effective.

3.2.2 Vertebral tethering techniques

VBT is a recent compression-based implant technique introduced by Crawford et al. [74]. It involves the thoracoscopic placement of anterior vertebral body screw anchors with a tightened flexible tether between them. This method achieves correction through both tether tension and spinal translation, all performed via an endoscopic approach.

Indications for VBT include thoracic curves within the range of 30°–70° and thoracolumbar or lumbar curves ranging from 30° to 60° in skeletally immature patients. However, the presence of hyperkyphosis (>40°) in the thoracic region is considered a relative contraindication due to the use of anterior instrumentation [36].

In a study conducted by Samdani et al. thoracic curve correction was reported in 32 patients, reducing from an average of 42.8°–21.0° on the initial erect radiograph and 17.9° at the latest follow-up. Additionally, the non-instrumented lumbar curve exhibited significant spontaneous correction, decreasing from 25° to 18° at the first follow-up and 13° at the final follow-up [75]. In Hoernschemeyer et al. [76] presented the results of a study involving skeletally immature patients treated with VBT, achieving a success rate of 74% in attaining curve magnitudes less than 30° at skeletal maturity.

In summary, VBT represents a promising approach for correcting certain spinal deformities in skeletally immature patients, demonstrating favorable outcomes in select cases.

3.3 Guided growth systems

3.3.1 Luque trolley technique

The Luque trolley technique utilizes sublaminar wires to segmentally fix rods to the spine, aiming to limit subperiosteal dissection to prevent unintentional spinal fusion [29]. However, this approach is not commonly employed due to documented issues such as spontaneous spinal fusion, limited spinal growth, and control of spinal deformity [77].

A more recent development is the Modern Luque Trolley (MLT) system, introduced by Ouellet et al., who published a 5-year retrospective study involving five patients. The study showed that MLT successfully corrected primary curves, reducing them from 60 to 21°, with the maintenance of correction observed during a 2-year follow-up period. Notably, MLT does not rely on sublaminar or cerclage wires. Instead, it employs gliding spinal anchors that travel along fixed, overlapping rods. This technique can effectively halt the progression of spinal deformities while still allowing for relatively normal spinal growth. While concerns about spinal fusion may persist, the study reported fewer implant failures compared to the original trolley technique [78].

Indications for MLT include a Cobb angle exceeding 40°, failed conservative treatment, and significant growth potential [79]. It is important to note that MLT is a relatively new technique and has yet to receive official approval in many regions.

In summary, MLT represents a promising advancement in the treatment of spinal deformities, addressing some of the limitations associated with traditional Luque trolley methods.

3.3.2 Shilla technique

The Shilla technique, introduced by McCarthy and colleagues [80], represents a relatively recent procedure that adheres to the growth principles of guided growth systems. It involves the fixation of dual rods using pedicle screws at the apex of the spinal curve, with proximal and distal gliding screws employed to minimize subperiosteal dissection, thereby preventing spontaneous fusion at these segments [35].

In the Shilla technique, the initial correction focuses on the apical deformity, aligning it toward a neutral position. Subsequently, the upper and lower growth guidance segments extend into the distal and proximal regions of the curve using polyaxial screws. These specialized screws feature locking caps that attach to the top of the screws (rather than the rod), capturing the rod and allowing it to slide longitudinally with growth. This approach eliminates the need for multiple open lengthening surgeries similar to MCGRs. Present indications for the Shilla technique include cases where bracing has proven ineffective and when dealing with coronal curves exceeding 50° [80].

In McCarthy et al. [81] reported findings from a study involving 40 patients with a minimum 5-year follow-up, encompassing various scoliosis types (nine idiopathic, one congenital, 16 neuromuscular, and 14 syndromic). The average preoperative curve measured 69°, which was reduced to 25° following the index procedures, and at the most recent follow-up or prior to definitive spinal fusion, the curve averaged 38.4°.

In Luhmann et al. [82] compared the Shilla technique and TGRs radiographically. They observed that preoperative curves with mean values of 61° and 65° in the two groups had corrected to 27° and 29°, respectively, at the latest follow-up. The growth of the T1–T12 segment increased by 4.6 cm for the Shilla technique and 5.2 cm for TGR. Both methods demonstrated favorable radiographic outcomes regarding growth, curve correction, and complications. A notable distinction was the Shilla technique's threefold reduction in overall surgeries.

However, despite the advantage of reducing the total number of surgeries, concerns about complication rates, particularly implant-related complications, persist similar to MCGR and TGR. These complications have been reported to reach as high as 73%, leading to return surgeries due to secondary infections, alignment issues, and implant-related problems [81]. Wilkinson et al. [83] noted that the apex of the fused primary curve shifted in approximately 62% of patients, with nearly all of these cases (92%) involving distal migration.

In summary, the Shilla technique is a promising approach for spinal deformity correction, showing advantages in terms of reduced surgeries compared to TGRs. However, complications, especially implant-related problems, remain a significant concern, and long-term studies are needed to better assess its effectiveness and safety.

3.4 Other alternatives

3.4.1 Vertebral column resection

Vertebrectomy for severe scoliosis was initially introduced by MacLennan [84]. Over time, this technique has evolved into vertebral column resection (VCR), which now involves a three-column circumferential osteotomy encompassing the vertebral body, adjacent disks, pedicles, and all dorsal elements. This creates a segmental defect, inducing instability and necessitating provisional instrumentation [85].

Current indications for VCR mainly involve addressing short angular deformities, especially in cases where other methods are technically unfeasible, often seen in congenital scoliosis (CS) or early-onset congenital kyphosis [86]. Hemivertebrae, a common pathology in CS, often results in a wedge-shaped deformity that progresses with spinal growth. Hemivertebrae resection has emerged as the gold standard treatment for CS caused by hemivertebrae, yielding excellent curve correction results [87].

Traditionally, this procedure was performed via an anterior-posterior approach. However, due to prolonged operative times, substantial blood loss, and elevated complication rates, there has been a shift toward adopting a posterolateral approach more recently [86]. Despite improvements in surgical duration and blood loss with this approach, concerns persist regarding its technical complexity, potential blood loss, and heightened complication rates, especially concerning neurologic complications. Therefore, when considering VCR, it should be cautiously approached by an experienced surgical team [85].

A study by Wang and Zhang [88] focused on 36 CS patients (mean age: 59 months; mean follow-up: 62.3 months) with hemivertebrae who underwent hemivertebra resection and segmental fusion. They achieved significant correction of segmental scoliosis (from 36.6° to 5.1°) and segmental kyphosis (from 21.2° to 5.8°) at the last follow-up. Complications included one case of delayed wound healing, two cases of pedicle fractures, and one case of progressive deformity. These patients, typically very young with poor bone quality and thin, soft tissue coverage, face higher risks of wound healing issues and screw displacements than adults. However, satisfactory outcomes and prognoses can be achieved with careful management, malformation correction, and solid fusion.

In summary, VCR is valuable for addressing severe scoliosis and congenital spinal deformities. It is especially effective in cases of hemivertebrae-related deformities, although it comes with potential complications, requiring a skilled surgical team for optimal outcomes.

3.4.2 Convex hemiepiphysiodesis

Convex hemiepiphysiodesis, also referred to as convex growth arrest, was once a commonly employed technique for managing congenital scoliosis in children [89]. This method was primarily used to address multilevel congenital deformities, and while it was considered safe and straightforward, its ability to guide and regulate spinal growth was somewhat unpredictable [90].

In a 2020 study by Rizkallah et al. [89], 22 patients with congenital scoliosis underwent a 1-staged double approach hemiepiphysiodesis involving bone grafting of the convex side without instrumentation. The study concluded that limited convex hemiepiphysiodesis remains a viable option in the treatment of congenital scoliosis, especially in patients ≤3 years old, with curves ≤35°, and isolated hemivertebra. This approach offers certain advantages, sparing patients the risks associated with vertebral resection and instrumentation while achieving fusion across the same number of levels.

4. Future directions

The current approach to treating EOS prioritizes addressing spinal and thoracic cage deformities, improving cardiopulmonary function, addressing psychological impact and enhancing health-related quality of life. Over recent years, substantial advancements have been in comprehending EOS's natural progression and long-term consequences. Moreover, technological innovations have expanded the treatment options available to EOS patients. However, despite these advances, EOS remains a complex challenge, marked by a lack of consensus among experts in the field [91]. The proliferation of treatment options has outpaced the availability of evidence-based literature, leading to uncertainties in managing EOS effectively. Additionally, various obstacles hinder the acquisition of high-level evidence in EOS treatment. These obstacles include the small and diverse patient population, the need for extended follow-up periods, the absence of reliable prognostic classifications, and the difficulties in assessing pulmonary outcomes in this specific patient group.

Classification systems serve as crucial tools in healthcare, allowing the characterization of medical conditions, suggesting potential prognoses, and guiding treatment decisions. However, a significant challenge arises when it comes to early-onset scoliosis (EOS)—the existing classification systems are not reliably prognostic. This issue highlights the pressing need for further research in this field to enhance the utility of classification systems in identifying trends of successful and unsuccessful treatment options for EOS patients. To address this limitation and improve the efficacy of EOS treatment, the integration of artificial intelligence (AI) holds significant promise. With its remarkable ability in data analysis and pattern recognition, AI can help create more practical and accurate classifications for EOS. By leveraging AI algorithms, classification systems can be refined to categorize EOS cases and predict their likely treatment outcomes. Furthermore, the application of AI in EOS research can benefit from big data and multicentric studies. Gathering extensive patient data from various medical centers and incorporating it into AI-driven analyses can lead to more comprehensive and accurate classification systems. This approach ensures that a narrow dataset does not limit classification systems but encompasses a diverse range of EOS cases.

Although evidence supports the effectiveness of treatments in correcting spinal curvature and promoting spinal growth in early-onset scoliosis (EOS), concerns persist regarding their impact on enhancing pulmonary function. It has become evident that conventional radiographic assessments are insufficient for adequately gauging respiratory outcomes in EOS patients. The development of advanced imaging techniques capable of providing three-dimensional dynamic measurements, in conjunction with other assessment modalities, holds the potential to enhance our understanding of pulmonary outcomes in children undergoing treatment. These advancements are promising in improving the evaluation of the intricate relationship between the spine, thorax, and pulmonary function. Progress in these areas is crucial because it can lead to a more comprehensive understanding of how to prevent the progression of EOS to thoracic insufficiency syndrome (TIS), which ultimately results in cardiopulmonary compromise [92, 93].

5. Conclusion

EOS encompasses a spectrum of spinal growth pathologies with diverse causes and presentations, demanding a multifaceted approach to treatment. Successful management should prioritize the correction of spinal and thoracic cage deformities, enhancing respiratory function, and improving health-related quality of life for affected children. Addressing EOS poses significant challenges, with treatment strategies necessitating tailored approaches considering the specific deformity type, underlying causes, and potential coexisting medical conditions. Despite our abundant knowledge of EOS, it remains a condition without a definitive, one-size-fits-all solution. The early identification and accurate classification of EOS are of utmost importance in providing effective treatment strategies. Each case warrants a personalized plan tailored to its unique characteristics and underlying etiology. Conservative treatments should be explored as the initial course of action whenever possible.

Recent advancements have spurred growing interest in applying Mehta's casting method for treating idiopathic scoliosis. This promising approach is gaining recognition and acceptance within the medical community as an effective treatment option for idiopathic cases, showcasing its potential to provide positive patient outcomes. For other cases, a meticulous and multidisciplinary approach is indispensable. A dedicated team of healthcare professionals, including pediatricians, nutritionists, physiotherapists, orthopedic specialists, and orthotics experts, must work collaboratively in managing these complex cases. This comprehensive approach acknowledges that scoliosis often accompanies other health concerns in children, necessitating holistic care that addresses various facets of their well-being.

Recognizing that spinal deformity represents just one aspect of a child's broader health issues is crucial. Therefore, comprehensive care should encompass all aspects of their physical, medical, and developmental needs. This multidisciplinary approach empowers healthcare providers to provide the highest quality of care and support for children with scoliosis, addressing their spinal health and overall well-being.

Moving forward, future efforts should prioritize technological advancements and treatment refinement. These include the development of prognostic classifications, enhancing pulmonary function assessment methodologies, conducting high-level clinical research, and ultimately improving the quality of life for EOS patients.

Acknowledgements

This research received no specific grant from funding agencies in the public, commercial, or not-for-profit sectors.

Conflict of interest

The authors declare no conflict of interest.

Author details

Hossein Nematian[1], Andrew Clarke[2*], Zahra Vahdati[1], Mohammad Hossein Nabian[1,3*] and Saeed Reza Mehrpour[3]

1 Center of Orthopedic Trans-Disciplinary Applied Research (COTAR), Tehran University of Medical Sciences, Tehran, Iran

2 Princess Elizabeth Orthopaedic Centre, Exeter, United Kingdom

3 Department of Orthopaedic and Trauma Surgery, Shariati Hospital, Tehran University of Medical Sciences, Tehran, Iran

*Address all correspondence to: andrewjsclarke@gmail.com and dr.nabian@gmail.com

References

[1] Ponseti IV, Friedman B. Prognosis in idiopathic scoliosis. The Journal of Bone and Joint Surgery. American Volume. 1950;**32a**(2):381-395

[2] James JI, Lloyd-Roberts GC, Pilcher MF. Infantile structural scoliosis. Journal of Bone and Joint Surgery. British Volume (London). 1959;**41-b**:719-735

[3] Dickson RA. Conservative treatment for idiopathic scoliosis. Journal of Bone and Joint Surgery. British Volume (London). 1985;**67**(2):176-181

[4] Weinstein SL, Wenger DR. The pediatric spine: Principles and practice. Journal of Pediatric Orthopaedics. 1994;**14**(5):680

[5] El-Hawary R, Akbarnia BA. Early onset scoliosis - Time for consensus. Spinal Deformity. 2015;**3**(2):105-106

[6] Williams BA, Matsumoto H, McCalla DJ, Akbarnia BA, Blakemore LC, Betz RR, et al. Development and initial validation of the classification of early-onset scoliosis (C-EOS). The Journal of Bone and Joint Surgery. American Volume. 2014;**96**(16):1359-1367

[7] Scott JC, Morgan TH. The natural history and prognosis of infantile idiopathic scoliosis. Journal of Bone and Joint Surgery. British Volume (London). 1955;**37-b**(3):400-413

[8] Pehrsson K, Larsson S, Oden A, Nachemson A. Long-term follow-up of patients with untreated scoliosis. A study of mortality, causes of death, and symptoms. Spine (Phila Pa) 1976. 1992;**17**(9):1091-1096

[9] Karol LA, Johnston C, Mladenov K, Schochet P, Walters P, Browne RH. Pulmonary function following early thoracic fusion in non-neuromuscular scoliosis. The Journal of Bone and Joint Surgery. American Volume. 2008;**90**(6):1272-1281

[10] Branthwaite MA. Cardiorespiratory consequences of unfused idiopathic scoliosis. British Journal of Diseases of the Chest. 1986;**80**(4):360-369

[11] Dimeglio A. Growth in pediatric orthopedics. In: Morrissy RT, Weinstein SL, editors. Lovell and Winter's Pediatric Orthopaedics. 6th ed. Philadelphia: Lippincott Williams & Wilkins; 2006

[12] Helenius IJ. Normal and Abnormal Growth of Spine. Non-Idiopathic Spine Deformities in Young Children. Berlin, Heidelberg: Springer; 2011. pp. 3-13

[13] Schittny JC. Development of the lung. Cell and Tissue Research. 2017;**367**(3):427-444

[14] Canavese F, Dimeglio A. Normal and abnormal spine and thoracic cage development. World Journal of Orthopedics. 2013;**4**(4):167-174

[15] Davies G, Reid L. Effect of scoliosis on growth of alveoli and pulmonary arteries and on right ventricle. Archives of Disease in Childhood. 1971;**46**(249):623-632

[16] Johnston CE, Karol LA, Thornberg D, Jo C, Eamara P. The 18-cm thoracic-height threshold and pulmonary function in non-neuromuscular early-onset scoliosis: A reassessment. JB JS Open Access. 2021;**6**(4):e21.00093

[17] Cunin V. Early-onset scoliosis: Current treatment. Orthopaedics &

Traumatology, Surgery & Research. 2015;**101**(1 Suppl):S109-S118

[18] Yang S, Andras LM, Redding GJ, Skaggs DL. Early-onset scoliosis: A review of history, current treatment, and future directions. Pediatrics. 2016;**137**(1)

[19] Xu E, Gao R, Jiang H, Lin T, Shao W, Zhou X. Combined halo gravity traction and dual growing rod technique for the treatment of early onset dystrophic scoliosis in Neurofibromatosis type 1. World Neurosurgery. 2019;**126**:e173-ee80

[20] Welborn MC, Krajbich JI, D'Amato C. Use of magnetic spinal growth rods (MCGR) with and without preoperative halo-gravity traction (HGT) for the treatment of severe early-onset scoliosis (EOS). Journal of Pediatric Orthopedics. 2019;**39**(4):e293-e2e7

[21] Iyer S, Duah HO, Wulff I, Osei Tutu H, Mahmud R, Yankey KP, et al. The use of halo gravity traction in the treatment of severe early onset spinal deformity. Spine (Phila Pa 1976). 2019;**44**(14):E841-E8e5

[22] Baulesh DM, Huh J, Judkins T, Garg S, Miller NH, Erickson MA. The role of serial casting in early-onset scoliosis (EOS). Journal of Pediatric Orthopedics. 2012;**32**(7):658-663

[23] Fletcher ND, McClung A, Rathjen KE, Denning JR, Browne R, Johnston CE 3rd. Serial casting as a delay tactic in the treatment of moderate-to-severe early-onset scoliosis. Journal of Pediatric Orthopedics. 2012;**32**(7):664-671

[24] Sanders JO, D'Astous J, Fitzgerald M, Khoury JG, Kishan S, Sturm PF. Derotational casting for progressive infantile scoliosis. Journal of Pediatric Orthopedics. 2009;**29**(6):581-587

[25] Mehta MH. Growth as a corrective force in the early treatment of progressive infantile scoliosis. Journal of Bone and Joint Surgery. British Volume (London). 2005;**87**(9):1237-1247

[26] Gussous YM, Tarima S, Zhao S, Khan S, Caudill A, Sturm P, et al. Serial Derotational casting in idiopathic and non-idiopathic progressive early-onset scoliosis. Spinal Deformity. 2015;**3**(3):233-238

[27] Iorio J, Orlando G, Diefenbach C, Gaughan JP, Samdani AF, Pahys JM, et al. Serial casting for infantile idiopathic scoliosis: Radiographic outcomes and factors associated with response to treatment. Journal of Pediatric Orthopedics. 2017;**37**(5):311-316

[28] Ballhause TM, Moritz M, Hättich A, Stücker R, Mladenov K. Serial casting in early onset scoliosis: Syndromic scoliosis is no contraindication. BMC Musculoskeletal Disorders. 2019;**20**(1):554

[29] Beauchamp EC, Anderson RCE, Vitale MG. Modern surgical management of early onset and adolescent idiopathic scoliosis. Neurosurgery. 2019;**84**(2):291-304

[30] Weinstein SL, Dolan LA, Wright JG, Dobbs MB. Effects of bracing in adolescents with idiopathic scoliosis. The New England Journal of Medicine. 2013;**369**(16):1512-1521

[31] Thometz J, Liu XC. Serial CAD/CAM bracing: An alternative to serial casting for early onset scoliosis. Journal of Pediatric Orthopedics. 2019;**39**(3):e185-e1e9

[32] Thometz J, Liu X, Rizza R, English I, Tarima S. Effect of an elongation bending derotation brace on the infantile or juvenile scoliosis. Scoliosis and Spinal Disorders. 2018;**13**:13

[33] Smith JR, Samdani AF, Pahys J, Ranade A, Asghar J, Cahill P, et al. The role of bracing, casting, and vertical expandable prosthetic titanium rib for the treatment of infantile idiopathic scoliosis: A single-institution experience with 31 consecutive patients. Clinical article. Journal of Neurosurgery: Spine. 2009;**11**(1):3-8

[34] Teoh KH, Winson DM, James SH, Jones A, Howes J, Davies PR, et al. Do magnetic growing rods have lower complication rates compared with conventional growing rods? The Spine Journal. 2016;**16**(4 Suppl):S40-S44

[35] Skaggs DL, Akbarnia BA, Flynn JM, Myung KS, Sponseller PD, Vitale MG. A classification of growth friendly spine implants. Journal of Pediatric Orthopedics. 2014;**34**(3):260-274

[36] Hardesty CK, Huang RP, El-Hawary R, Samdani A, Hermida PB, Bas T, et al. Early-onset scoliosis: Updated treatment techniques and results. Spinal Deformity. 2018;**6**(4):467-472

[37] Harrington PR. Treatment of scoliosis. Correction and internal fixation by spine instrumentation. The Journal of Bone and Joint Surgery. American Volume. 1962;**44-a**:591-610

[38] Moe JH, Kharrat K, Winter RB, Cummine JL. Harrington instrumentation without fusion plus external orthotic support for the treatment of difficult curvature problems in young children. Clinical Orthopaedics and Related Research. 1984;**185**:35-45

[39] Mineiro J, Weinstein SL. Subcutaneous rodding for progressive spinal curvatures: Early results. Journal of Pediatric Orthopedics. 2002;**22**(3):290-295

[40] Akbarnia BA, Marks DS, Boachie-Adjei O, Thompson AG, Asher MA. Dual growing rod technique for the treatment of progressive early-onset scoliosis: A multicenter study. Spine (Phila Pa 1976). 2005;**30**(17 Suppl):S46-S57

[41] Yang JS, McElroy MJ, Akbarnia BA, Salari P, Oliveira D, Thompson GH, et al. Growing rods for spinal deformity: Characterizing consensus and variation in current use. Journal of Pediatric Orthopedics. 2010;**30**(3):264-270

[42] Bess S, Akbarnia BA, Thompson GH, Sponseller PD, Shah SA, El Sebaie H, et al. Complications of growing-rod treatment for early-onset scoliosis: Analysis of one hundred and forty patients. The Journal of Bone and Joint Surgery. American Volume. 2010;**92**(15):2533-2543

[43] Sankar WN, Acevedo DC, Skaggs DL. Comparison of complications among growing spinal implants. Spine (Phila Pa 1976). 2010;**35**(23):2091-2096

[44] Akbarnia BA, Breakwell LM, Marks DS, McCarthy RE, Thompson AG, Canale SK, et al. Dual growing rod technique followed for three to eleven years until final fusion: The effect of frequency of lengthening. Spine (Phila Pa 1976). 2008;**33**(9):984-990

[45] Nematian H, Clarke A, Hedayat E, Vahdati Z, Milan N, Mehrpour SR, et al. Complications of single growing rod constructs in the treatment of severe early-onset scoliosis: A lesson relearned. Spinal Deformity. 2022;**10**(6):1481-1490

[46] Shah SA, Karatas AF, Dhawale AA, Dede O, Mundis GM Jr, Holmes L Jr, et al. The effect of serial growing rod lengthening on the sagittal profile and pelvic parameters in early-onset scoliosis. Spine (Phila Pa 1976). 2014;**39**(22):E1311-E1317

[47] Watanabe K, Uno K, Suzuki T, Kawakami N, Tsuji T, Yanagida H, et al. Risk factors for proximal junctional kyphosis associated with dual-rod growing-rod surgery for early-onset scoliosis. Clinical Spine Surgery. 2016;**29**(8):E428-E433

[48] Thompson GH, Akbarnia BA, Kostial P, Poe-Kochert C, Armstrong DG, Roh J, et al. Comparison of single and dual growing rod techniques followed through definitive surgery: A preliminary study. Spine (Phila Pa 1976). 2005;**30**(18):2039-2044

[49] Xu G-J, Fu X, Tian P, Ma J-X, Ma X-L. Comparison of single and dual growing rods in the treatment of early onset scoliosis: A meta-analysis. Journal of Orthopaedic Surgery and Research. 2016;**11**(1):80

[50] Luhmann SJ, Skaggs DL, Pahys J, Samdani A, El-Hawary R. Single distraction-rod constructs in severe early-onset scoliosis: Indications and outcomes. The Spine Journal. 2021;**22**(2):305-312

[51] Hickey BA, Towriss C, Baxter G, Yasso S, James S, Jones A, et al. Early experience of MAGEC magnetic growing rods in the treatment of early onset scoliosis. European Spine Journal. 2014;**23 Suppl 1**(Suppl. 1):S61-S65

[52] La Rosa G, Oggiano L, Ruzzini L. Magnetically controlled growing rods for the Management of Early-onset Scoliosis: A preliminary report. Journal of Pediatric Orthopedics. 2017;**37**(2):79-85

[53] Akbarnia BA, Cheung K, Noordeen H, Elsebaie H, Yazici M, Dannawi Z, et al. Next generation of growth-sparing techniques: Preliminary clinical results of a magnetically controlled growing rod in 14 patients with early-onset scoliosis. Spine (Phila Pa 1976). 2013;**38**(8):665-670

[54] Akbarnia BA, Pawelek JB, Cheung KM, Demirkiran G, Elsebaie H, Emans JB, et al. Traditional growing rods versus magnetically controlled growing rods for the surgical treatment of early-onset scoliosis: A case-matched 2-year study. Spinal Deformity. 2014;**2**(6):493-497

[55] Aslan C, Olgun ZD, Ayik G, Karaokur R, Ozusta S, Demirkiran GH, et al. Does decreased surgical stress really improve the psychosocial health of early-onset scoliosis patients?: A comparison of traditional growing rods and magnetically-controlled growing rods patients reveals disappointing results. Spine (Phila Pa 1976). 2019;**44**(11):E656-Ee63

[56] Doany ME, Olgun ZD, Kinikli GI, Bekmez S, Kocyigit A, Demirkiran G, et al. Health-related quality of life in early-onset scoliosis patients treated surgically: EOSQ scores in traditional growing rod versus magnetically controlled growing rods. Spine (Phila Pa 1976). 2018;**43**(2):148-153

[57] Kwan KYH, Alanay A, Yazici M, Demirkiran G, Helenius I, Nnadi C, et al. Unplanned reoperations in magnetically controlled growing rod surgery for early onset scoliosis with a minimum of two-year follow-up. Spine (Phila Pa 1976). 2017;**42**(24):E1410-E14e4

[58] Baky FJ, Larson AN, St Hilaire T, Pawelek J, Skaggs DL, Emans JB, et al. The effect of expansion thoracostomy on spine growth in patients with spinal deformity and fused ribs treated with rib-based growing constructs. Spinal Deformity. 2019;**7**(5):836-841

[59] Campbell RM Jr, Smith MD, Hell-Vocke AK. Expansion thoracoplasty: The surgical technique of opening-wedge thoracostomy. Surgical technique. The Journal of Bone and Joint Surgery. American Volume. 2004;**86** (A Suppl. 1):51-64

[60] Yazici M, Emans J. Fusionless instrumentation systems for congenital scoliosis: Expandable spinal rods and vertical expandable prosthetic titanium rib in the management of congenital spine deformities in the growing child. Spine (Phila Pa 1976). 2009;**34**(17):1800-1807

[61] Hasler CC, Mehrkens A, Hefti F. Efficacy and safety of VEPTR instrumentation for progressive spine deformities in young children without rib fusions. European Spine Journal. 2010;**19**(3):400-408

[62] Ramirez N, Camacho L, Ibanez M, Ramirez N, Torres Y, Montanez J, et al. Respiratory and Postoperative Outcomes in Early Onset Scoliosis Patients Treated with Rib Based Growing System: Single Centre Experience of 15 Years. IL, USA: American Academy of Pediatrics Itasca; 2021

[63] Waldhausen JH, Redding G, White K, Song K. Complications in using the vertical expandable prosthetic titanium rib (VEPTR) in children. Journal of Pediatric Surgery. 2016;**51**(11):1747-1750

[64] Campbell RM Jr, Smith MD, Mayes TC, Mangos JA, Willey-Courand DB, Kose N, et al. The effect of opening wedge thoracostomy on thoracic insufficiency syndrome associated with fused ribs and congenital scoliosis. The Journal of Bone and Joint Surgery. American Volume. 2004;**86**(8):1659-1674

[65] Ramirez N, Olivella G, Rodriguez O, Marrero P, Smith J, Garg S, et al. Incidence of complications in the management of non-ambulatory neuromuscular early-onset scoliosis with a rib-based growing system: High- versus low-tone patients. European Journal of Orthopaedic Surgery and Traumatology. 2020;**30**(4):621-627

[66] Stokes IA. Mechanical effects on skeletal growth. Journal of Musculoskeletal & Neuronal Interactions. 2002;**2**(3):277-280

[67] Nachlas IW, Borden JN. The cure of experimental scoliosis by directed growth control. The Journal of Bone and Joint Surgery. American Volume. 1951; **33 a**(1):24-34

[68] Smith AD, Von Lackum WH, Wylie R. An operation for stapling vertebral bodies in congenital scoliosis. The Journal of Bone and Joint Surgery. American Volume. 1954;**36**(A:2):342-348

[69] Guille JT, D'Andrea LP, Betz RR. Fusionless treatment of scoliosis. The Orthopedic Clinics of North America. 2007;**38**(4):541-545

[70] Trobisch PD, Samdani A, Cahill P, Betz RR. Vertebral body stapling as an alternative in the treatment of idiopathic scoliosis. Operative Orthopädie und Traumatologie. 2011;**23**(3):227-231

[71] Betz RR, Kim J, D'Andrea LP, Mulcahey MJ, Balsara RK, Clements DH. An innovative technique of vertebral body stapling for the treatment of patients with adolescent idiopathic scoliosis: A feasibility, safety, and utility study. Spine (Phila Pa 1976). 2003;**28**(20):S255-S265

[72] Bumpass DB, Fuhrhop SK, Schootman M, Smith JC, Luhmann SJ. Vertebral body stapling for moderate juvenile and early adolescent idiopathic scoliosis: Cautions and patient selection criteria. Spine (Phila Pa 1976). 2015;**40**(24):E1305-E1314

[73] Cahill PJ, Auriemma M, Dakwar E, Gaughan JP, Samdani AF, Pahys JM, et al. Factors predictive of outcomes in vertebral body stapling for idiopathic scoliosis. Spinal Deformity. 2018;**6**(1):28-37

[74] Crawford CH 3rd, Lenke LG. Growth modulation by means of anterior tethering resulting in progressive correction of juvenile idiopathic scoliosis: A case report. The Journal of Bone and Joint Surgery. American Volume. 2010;**92**(1):202-209

[75] Samdani AF, Ames RJ, Kimball JS, Pahys JM, Grewal H, Pelletier GJ, et al. Anterior vertebral body tethering for immature adolescent idiopathic scoliosis: One-year results on the first 32 patients. European Spine Journal. 2015;**24**(7):1533-1539

[76] Hoernschemeyer DG, Boeyer ME, Robertson ME, Loftis CM, Worley JR, Tweedy NM, et al. Anterior vertebral body tethering for adolescent scoliosis with growth remaining: A retrospective review of 2 to 5-year postoperative results. The Journal of Bone and Joint Surgery. American Volume. 2020;**102**(13):1169-1176

[77] Pratt RK, Webb JK, Burwell RG, Cummings SL. Luque trolley and convex epiphysiodesis in the management of infantile and juvenile idiopathic scoliosis. Spine (Phila Pa 1976). 1999;**24**(15):1538-1547

[78] Ouellet J. Surgical technique: Modern Luqué trolley, a self-growing rod technique. Clinical Orthopaedics and Related Research. 2011;**469**(5):1356-1367

[79] Alkhalife YI, Padhye KP, El-Hawary R. New technologies in pediatric spine surgery. The Orthopedic Clinics of North America. 2019;**50**(1):57-76

[80] McCarthy RE, Luhmann S, Lenke L, McCullough FL. The Shilla growth guidance technique for early-onset spinal deformities at 2-year follow-up: A preliminary report. Journal of Pediatric Orthopedics. 2014;**34**(1):1-7

[81] McCarthy RE, McCullough FL. Shilla growth guidance for early-onset scoliosis: Results after a minimum of five years of follow-up. The Journal of Bone and Joint Surgery. American Volume. 2015;**97**(19):1578-1584

[82] Luhmann SJ, Smith JC, McClung A, McCullough FL, McCarthy RE, Thompson GH. Radiographic outcomes of Shilla growth guidance system and traditional growing rods through definitive treatment. Spinal Deformity. 2017;**5**(4):277-282

[83] Wilkinson JT, Songy CE, Bumpass DB, McCullough FL, McCarthy RE. Curve modulation and apex migration using Shilla growth guidance rods for early-onset scoliosis at 5-year follow-up. Journal of Pediatric Orthopedics. 2019;**39**(8):400-405

[84] MacLennan A. Scoliosis. The British Medical Journal. 1922;**2**(3227):864-866

[85] Yang C, Zheng Z, Liu H, Wang J, Kim YJ, Cho S. Posterior vertebral column resection in spinal deformity: A systematic review. European Spine Journal. 2016;**25**(8):2368-2375

[86] Verma K, Slattery C, Duah H, Yankey KP, Mundis G, Boachie-Adjel O. Comprehensive assessment of outcomes from patients with severe early-onset scoliosis treated with a vertebral column resection: Results from an SRS global outreach site (FOCOS) in Ghana. Journal of Pediatric Orthopedics. 2018;**38**(7):e393-e3e8

[87] Jalanko T, Rintala R, Puisto V, Helenius I. Hemivertebra resection for congenital scoliosis in young children: Comparison of clinical, radiographic, and health-related quality of life outcomes between the anteroposterior and posterolateral approaches. Spine (Phila Pa 1976). 2011;**36**(1):41-49

[88] Wang S, Zhang J, Qiu G, Li S, Zhang Y, Yang Y, et al. Posterior-only hemivertebra resection with anterior structural reconstruction with titanium mesh cage and short segmental fusion for the treatment of congenital Scoliokyphosis: The indications and preliminary results. Spine (Phila Pa 1976). 2017;**42**(22):1687-1692

[89] Rizkallah M, Sebaaly A, Kharrat K, Kreichati G. Is there still a place for convex Hemiepiphysiodesis in congenital scoliosis in young children? A long-term follow-up. Global Spine Journal. 2020;**10**(4):406-411

[90] Alanay A, Dede O, Yazici M. Convex instrumented hemiepiphysiodesis with concave distraction: A preliminary report. Clinical Orthopaedics and Related Research. 2012;**470**(4):1144-1150

[91] Hughes MS, Swarup I, Makarewich CA, Williams BA, Talwar D, Cahill PJ, et al. Expert consensus for early onset scoliosis surgery. Journal of Pediatric Orthopedics. 2020;**40**(7):e621-e6e8

[92] Glotzbecker M, Johnston C, Miller P, Smith J, Perez-Grueso FS, Woon R, et al. Is there a relationship between thoracic dimensions and pulmonary function in early-onset scoliosis? Spine (Phila Pa 1976). 2014;**39**(19):1590-1595

[93] Campbell RM Jr, Smith MD, Mayes TC, Mangos JA, Willey-Courand DB, Kose N, et al. The characteristics of thoracic insufficiency syndrome associated with fused ribs and congenital scoliosis. The Journal of Bone and Joint Surgery. American Volume. 2003;**85**(3):399-408